INVINCIBLE LIVING

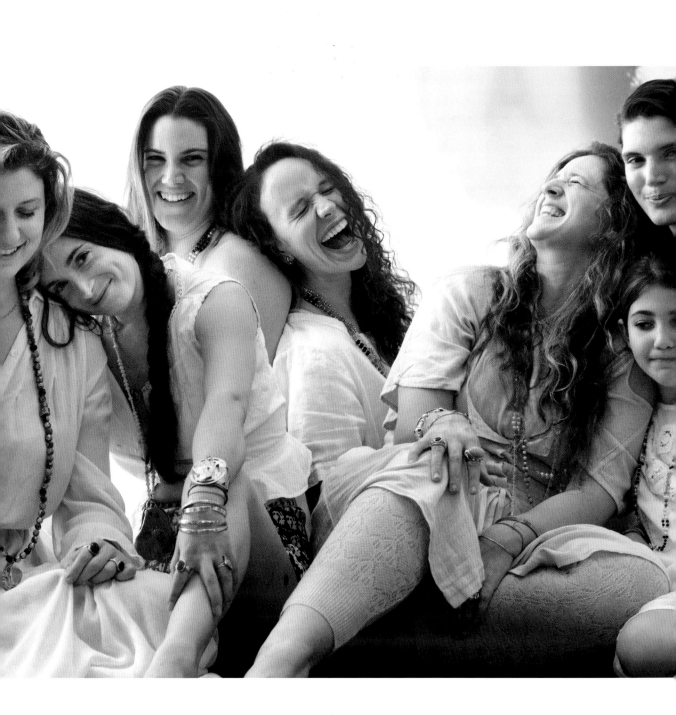

INVINCIBLE LIVING

THE POWER OF YOGA, THE ENERGY OF BREATH, AND OTHER TOOLS FOR A RADIANT LIFE

Guru Jagat

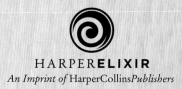

HARPER**ELIXIR**
An Imprint of HarperCollinsPublishers

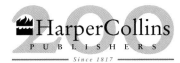

HarperCollins books may be purchased for educational, business, or sales promotional use. For information, please email the Special Markets Department at SPsales@harpercollins.com.

FIRST EDITION

Designed by Suet Yee Chong

Library of Congress Cataloging-in-Publication Data

Names: Jagat, Guru, author.
Title: Invincible living / by Guru Jagat.
Description: San Francisco : HarperElixir, [2017]
Identifiers: LCCN 2016028322 (print) | LCCN 2016044067 (ebook) |
ISBN 9780062414984 (hardcover) | ISBN 9780062415004 (e-book)
Subjects: LCSH: Kundalini.
Classification: LCC BL1238.56.K86 J34 2017 (print) |
LCC BL1238.56.K86 (ebook) | DDC 249.5/436—dc23
LC record available at https://lccn.loc.gov/2016028322.

17 18 19 20 21   QGT   10 9 8 7 6 5 4 3 2 1

This book is dedicated to the Golden Chain of Teachers,
Masters, and Artists who have given their lives, minds, bodies,
and art to the creation of beauty, kindness, compassion, and
the elevation of humankind. There are no words to express the
gratitude of the Great Treasures my Teachers Yogi Bhajan and
Harijiwan Khalsa have bestowed upon me. So I give this piece
of Dharma Art as an expression of this unending wave of Love
for what has been given to me so freely and generously.

Eternal gratitude to my deepest love John and dearest parents
Nansy, Rabbit, and Jamie. Thank you to Claudia, Libby, and the
amazing Harper Team as well Sharon Bowers extraordinaire.
Harmonjot you are a bright star and Shabadpreet and Julian thank
you for your ever present hard working loyal hearts. To Shane and all
the Gods de Love and Alive and Dead Poets Society—you poets are
my brothers and sisters. Immense gratitude to the people who put their
time, money, and energy on the line to support my vision and continue
to do so. Thank you so so so much. And lastly, this book is dedicated to
the RA MA community filled with stunning, awe-inspiring humans.

CONTENTS

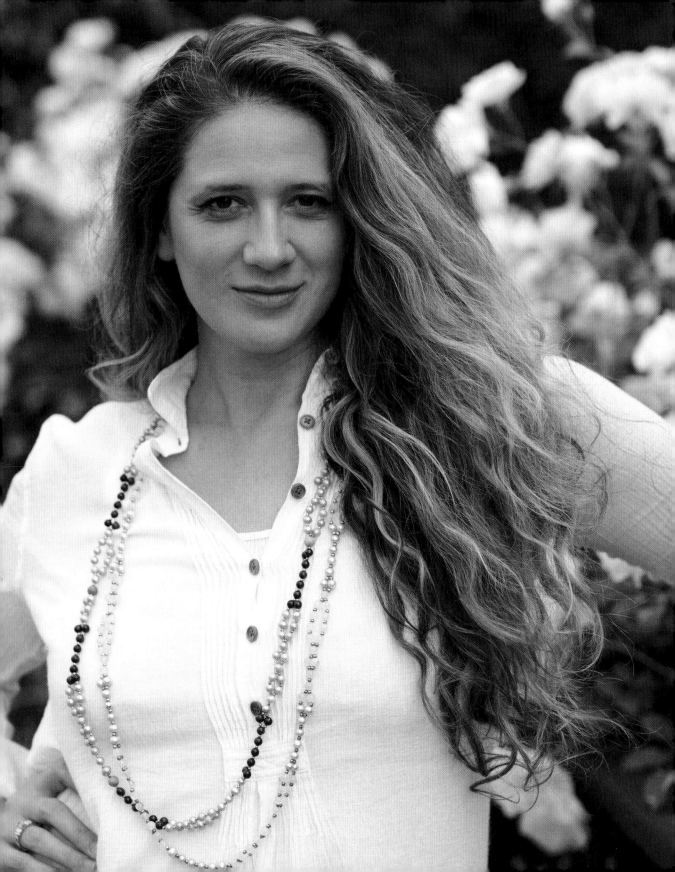

PREFACE

I am a modern woman, a yogi, a meditator, and in many ways my own version of a freedom fighter. I believe the new activism in this time is fighting for and freeing your mind, body, and emotions from the hypnotic media haze, denatured nutritional vitality suppression, and the general culturally accepted commotionality and subsequent fatigue we call "living a life." From a very early age I have been studying the lineages of Great Masters and Teachers who made their life an example of what was possible for humanity. I grew up in a struggling family with a single mother, trying to make ends meet—and at the same time all of us, my mother, brother, and I, were searching for community, spirituality, and creativity outside what religion was able to offer us. I was an avid questioner and seeker, and left no stone unturned to deepen my experience of questioning reality, my identity, and heightening creative expression through any means possible.

When I stumbled on the yoga scene that was happening in the early 2000s concurrently with some of my spiritual seeking, I was very put off by what felt to me, as a young person who came from a working-class background, to be self-centered and self-indulgent. It was similar to a lot of the spiritual scenes I was exposed to growing up—a lot of people concerned about a lot of themselves, their suffering, and ultimately their own neuroses. I vowed to myself to become an example of a deeply committed and spiritual person who on a daily basis was not drinking their own or anyone else's "Kool-Aid," as it were, that I would diligently and simply make my practice of infinity or spirituality about clearing myself enough of my own self-deception to be useful in any way to Society, to my family, and to anyone I came into contact with during the course of a day.

And then I came across Kundalini Yoga. It was post-911 New York City, and the whole collective consciousness had shifted dramatically. After twenty seconds of some weird arm-pumping posture, I had a *physical* experience of elevation and clarity that no other spiritual modality had even come close to touching. They all talked a lot about it. There was a lot of philosophy and rhetoric and theory about the elevation of human consciousness that I had listened to and read about over the years, but never had I had a real live experience of it so quickly and concisely in my own body.

I was practicing other forms of yoga for up to two hours a day at that point, and nothing like this had happened. Of course, I wanted to know more and experience more and I set out to practice as much as I could and go see the Master of this Lineage, Yogi Bhajan, at his ashram in New Mexico. He was still alive, and very sick at that point, but for two summers I was able to receive some direct transmissions of the experience of Kundalini Yoga and Meditation from him. How quick, effective, simple, and profound it is. It kept me hooked and wanting to learn and practice as much as I could.

I was very young at the time and didn't really know what I was doing or why, but had a keen sense of intuitive connection and a stubborn constitution that kept me glued to the path of discovering myself—my true Self—through the profound practices and tools of Kundalini Yoga. And what I have discovered over the years in my own practice and as a giver of these gifts that have been given to me is *how* to create a sustained, stable, elevated experience of human existence that is deeply fulfilling. The *how* is the most important part to me personally, because we are in an unprecedented time on the planet. Just as Yogi Bhajan predicted, now more than ever people need a *how* to quickly and efficiently remind them that there is something so much more profound and satisfying about life, love, relationships, work, creativity—about what we all crave as humans to experience more deeply.

For the past fifteen years, I have watched the pressure of the Technology Age consume more and more of our fading attention span and vitality. With it, the firsthand experience of how the demands we are facing as humans in a span of a day have exponentially increased with the skyrocketing technology. In this pressurization, something (many things) incredible has emerged, mainly a viral need for wellness on a deeper and deeper level; a quick and efficient way to release the pressure—more long lasting than a cocktail—an increased sensitivity to our interconnectedness as a planet, a galaxy, a star system; and the overwhelming momentum to find fulfillment as a human being that is not dependent on personal investment statistics, professional status, or what you look like.

The pressure is causing many people to look deeper into themselves to experience something more than the model of life stuck in a cycle of work, make money, have sex, have kids, travel a little, retire finally, and then get sick and die. To see that possibly there is a way to live that is more vital, more inspired, less based in fear and anxiety, and ultimately fulfilling for some deeper aspect of human life than survival of the fittest, war, competition, money, self-obsessed neurosis, and the suffering that a life full of turmoil creates on your physical, mental, and emotional well-being.

There is a different way. And you don't have to subscribe to any religion or touch your toes to experience it. You can—*right now*, in very little time—be connected to a deeper pulse of your life force, which manifests as instantaneous clarity, effectiveness, creativity, bravery, and the like. These are the pillars of Invincible Living, which are literally at your fingertips and take almost as much effort as picking up your smartphone. With the whole world, all information, and endless possibility available to you at the push of a button,

In this book I'll share with you my top yoga and lifestyle practices. One of the things that drew me to Kundalini Yoga is the spectrum of material from practical to esoteric that is available to learn, apply, and experience. Try these practices in an authentic way and see what truly works for you!

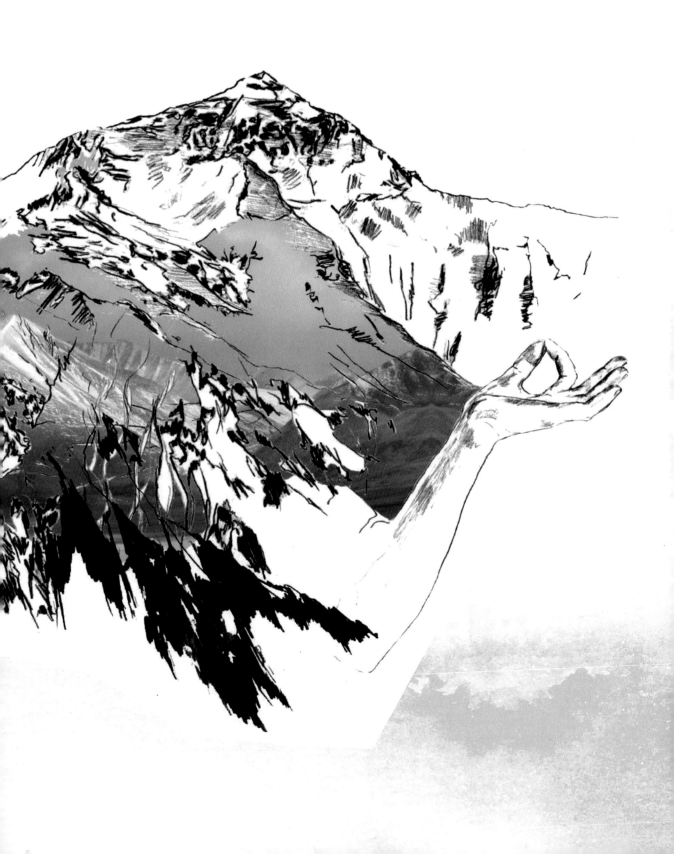

we all need something that will help us to navigate this increasingly complex experience on planet Earth.

And I'll tell you right now, I'm biased. After seeing so many people—people in the worst mental, physical, emotional states—people who might not make it another day, transform before my very eyes, I believe strongly in the quick and life-changing yogic and meditative technologies I'm offering to you in this book.

My own transformation has been profound, and every day I am reveling in the continued spark of more vitality, creative impulse, and just plain no-nonsense *joy* that I experience being alive. Now, that doesn't mean that there are not the ups and downs of a regular life, the losses and gains, the failures and successes. But what it does mean is that my mind and body have been trained to enjoy it all, to use whatever is in front of me as a way to know the great mystery of myself a little deeper.

And what is so fresh, so modern about these ancient Teachings is that they can touch anyone wherever they are in chronology, health, time demands, physical location, and so on. Kundalini Yoga and Meditation technologies are applicable to someone lying in a hospital bed, sitting in front of a computer, catching a self-care moment, or training as a professional or hobby athlete. We literally have eight thousand different techniques to prescriptively touch on every modern issue or need—quickly, without a barrier to entry and in a pair of jeans, high heels, athletic shoes, or no shoes at all. Yogi, meditator, professional, mom or dad, elderly, and athlete alike. The system is so complete, and most of the techniques take very little time.

And this alone is why I have committed my life to spreading these techniques. Because whether you choose to use pharmaceuticals, recreational drugs, shopping, sex, or the like to relieve some of this insistent consuming pressure on the human psyche and soma, I want you to know that there are other choices. And they're cheap, accessible, and take only a little bit of your time.

What takes *a lot* of time and energy is habitually trying to take the edge off of modern life with things that eventually leave you empty-handed. That includes the incessant fear of the future and habitually running from quieting ourselves for a moment, just enough to access some inherent human power called intuitive intelligence. There is burgeoning scientific research now proving the capacity of the human system to be aware, vital, and clear minded through the functioning of the multiple facets of the nervous system, biochemistry, and endocrine function, particularly the pituitary and pineal glands. And that the brains of meditators are literally physically structured differently and respond to stressors in a completely different way.

Yogis, sages, and meditators have recognized, experimented, and proven the strength, potential, and development of the human system for thousands of years. So these techniques are tried and true, and for over five thousand years they have been heavily practiced and proven to change your brain waves, chemistry, physical vitality, and thought patterns. Now, more than ever, the demand for these skills and choices is at a new peak. People of all walks of life, of all religious backgrounds, of all physical fitness levels, are flocking toward meditation and yoga as a way through the strongholds and pitfalls of our current daily human maladies and conditions.

So I offer you this book, from the heart of my Teachers and this profound Lineage through my own heart and practice, as a Choose Your Own Adventure into your own incredibly unique, distinguished, and breathtaking human dignity, intelligence, and grace. I offer these practices—from the most practical to the most esoteric, from stillness to movement—and this information as a way for you to empower your own deepest knowing and the forces of evolution and creativity that are moving uniquely through you in this *very* moment. Take some, leave some. Practice, breathe, give yourself a moment to explore the deeper parts of the mechanism of happiness and fulfillment that *are* inherent to you.

I promise you, this exploration will be one of the most valuable gifts you've ever given to yourself, your family, your business, your future, and the future of this planet.

Love and Awe, Guru Jagat

1. KUNDALINI YOGA Is for Everyone

Victory

According to current scientific theory, we waste 97 percent of our DNA. Most of our DNA is essentially trash, scientists argue, because we never turn it on, or even try to use it. These scientists honestly believe, through scientific reasoning, that we fail to tap into 97 percent of our DNA, literally 97 percent of our entire being—mind, body, and soul.

Leave it to modern science to throw out the stuff that we don't understand. As a yogic scientist, I believe that the 97 percent of our unused DNA is actually our human potential we have yet to turn on. The same with the brain. Most of us have activated only 3 percent of our brain, or, put another way, 3 percent of our total cerebral intelligence.

No matter how you say it, however—whether the brain is working and we're just not aware of it, or the brain is not working but it could be—we're still operating at only 3 percent. But we could be working with so much more. And I don't know about you, but I'm certainly interested in utilizing more of my inherent capacity as a human being—in energy, in intelligence, in creativity, and in possibility. This is exactly what Kundalini Yoga does, efficiently and effectively.

Your most amplified life is possible. That means amplified health, amplified happiness, amplified love, and amplified success. Yoga is a set of tools developed and refined over thousands of years that maximizes the body systems and the space-time continuum of the world around us, meaning our experience of reality, to create the most immense results in all areas of life. Kundalini Yoga is a pure, unbroken stream of these yogic practices and I believe is the quickest, most direct—and most accessible—way to activate your own path of Invincible Living.

There are no prerequisites for you to gain the benefits of Kundalini Yoga. No weights, no flexibility, no experience, no spirituality, no lexicon needed. Although if those things interest you or for some reason brought you to the mat, they absolutely can be found within the vast teachings of Kundalini Yoga. Likewise, you don't have to run off into a cave to meditate for twenty years. You can be you. In fact, these techniques uncover even more of your inherent essence, intelligence, and realness.

Known as a householder's tradition, Kundalini Yoga is for people with jobs, families, relationships, homes, cars, creative practices. In Kundalini Yoga, the path of ordinariness *is* the path to your own royalty, reality, and happiness. It's meant to give you—in the throes of changing diapers, changing jobs, getting married, getting divorced—enough energy to amplify all of those parts of your experience, so that regular life is invigorating and joyous. Meanwhile, it's a deeply meditative practice that can allow you to reach a so-called enlightened state or, to put it in a less intimidating way, a state of neutrality, even in the trenches of your everyday roles and responsibilities in the world.

Kundalini Yoga is *such* a powerful and useful practice for the modern world; it will quickly transform every aspect of your daily life. That's because Kundalini Yoga is for everyone. Anyone with a body, a mind, and a nervous system needs productive skills to cope with the pressures of the world. And it allows us to not just cope with these pressures but to succeed in the face of them. In this time of ever-increasing pressure and stress on the planet, I believe that yoga and meditative practice is no longer a luxury of people who have some extra time in their day or belong to a certain socioeconomic class.

CHANGE ON THE PLANET

We're in a new trajectory on the planet. This is a new time with new challenges, requirements, and rules of engagement than even five years ago. And part of what's happening is that the entire psychomagnetic field of the Earth is changing.

As a result of this shift in the Earth's psychomagnetic field, there's a pressure on our own *individual* psychomagnetic fields. Our own psyches, our own magnetic energies, have to change in order to keep up with the changes on the planet. The required upgrade is creating a very palpable pressure.

Whether we want to change or not, Kundalini Yoga is a technology that facilitates it. But as humans, there is within us a strong part of us that is afraid of and allergic to change. We go to great lengths to keep ourselves from being uncomfortable. But in our whole experience of life—the ebb and flow of it all—the friction of discomfort is exactly where the strengthening of ourselves, and deep self-fulfillment, actually occurs. This is why in Kundalini Yoga, we hold our arms up or our legs in certain ways or control the focus of our mind for periods of time. This is to *practice* being outside our energetic, physical, and psychoemotional comfort zones. It builds an unmistakable and unshakable strength.

With the demands of technology and the massive shifts in economic, geopolitical, and societal values that it's bringing, our human operating system is also upgrading. We have the choice to either consciously participate in this shift or be in conflict with it. Being in conflict with this upgrade is not unlike being in conflict about the upgrade on your phone. "I just don't have the time for the upgrade," we say when the notification pops up on our phone. "Stop asking me!" We push back the upgrade until later, again and again. But the upgrade has to happen for optimal functioning.

Kundalini Yoga is like the technology of your electronics, but it's for your biological and energetic/subtle bodies. The tech of Kundalini Yoga is that it allows you to relax, renew, and rejuvenate to such a degree that you are able to participate in elegance with the most mundane moments of every day. That may sound simple, but try it for one day—elegantly, gracefully, tolerantly move through every moment of your day. It takes a *huge* amount of fortitude, focus, and discipline.

WORKING FAST

What I love about the practices of Kundalini Yoga is that they can be so basic and still indescribably powerful. A little bit can go a long way. And the yoga works fast—as fast as the tech on your newest smartphone.

The pressure to evolve is so increased right now for humans that we don't have the leisure to take things slow. The planet is coming to a tipping point, and now more than ever we need people who are interested in cultivating a space within themselves that is still and interconnected to all that is. We need these people in every sector of society—people who have children, jobs, things they need to do, things to deliver in their respective areas of creativity . . . people who are *simultaneously* cultivating more tolerance, compassion, and understanding of themselves and others. It is said that using Hatha Yoga takes at a minimum twenty-two years to reach some level of mastery. Kundalini Yoga, on the other hand, is a tool of self-mastery, where the practitioner can reach major breakthroughs and exciting new heights within three minutes of practice. It's in no way qualitatively better than any other way, but it is certainly faster and works quickly no matter your physical, mental, emotional, and religious conditions.

A Vinyasa student once told me something really great about the Kundalini practice. She said, "You know, you put your arm up in this weird way and then you're breathing like crazy. You only do some postures on one side and it's totally nonlinear. But afterward—I just feel so much better!" We all just want and need something that's going to quickly give us a boost so that we can feel better.

Even Carl Jung, the great Swiss psychiatrist who founded analytical psychology, affirmed that the practices of Kundalini Yoga were far superior to anything he or Sigmund Freud were working on. He just didn't think that the world was ready for it. That was almost a hundred years ago. We are not only ready now, but we need it.

KUNDALINI YOGA FOR EVERYONE

There are a lot of barriers to entry in the yoga world, in my opinion, and they can seem to be in the Kundalini Yoga world too—a lot of mores and soft tones and unfamiliar words in other languages. One of my deepest, sincerest desires for you in your experience of this book is that you feel how *you* can pick up one or two of these practices that you enjoy, practice them for a couple of minutes, and have long-lasting, life-changing results. I find the yoga, meditation, and spiritual world to be a tricky place in the modern age because many of our high school cliché mentalities—consumerism, competitiveness, and tourism—leak into our inherent desire to feel better and touch something real in ourselves.

So no matching perfect spandex outfits required, no need to see yourself as spiritual or to know mantras or wear a *mala*, or to be *any* of those externalized versions of what a spiritual person, a yogi, or a meditator looks like. No need to get tripped up on the word *Kundalini* either. It's a wonderfully descriptive word that, in its sound, is describing this coiled potential literally within you. It is a fancy word that refers to your birthright, your wiring, your most activated version of yourself waiting for you in every moment, the happiest to the saddest—all the great and small moments that make up this incredible lifetime.

Kundalini just means "energy." Or, even less esoteric, *Kundalini* refers to a storehouse or power that's within all people regardless of age, gender, race, fitness level, or economic strata. And the technology of Kundalini Yoga is the physical, mental, and meditative practices that awaken and utilize that power.

Everybody on the planet right now is looking for some *experience of catharsis*. Whether it's with drugs or through music, this Technology Age pressure has created a numbness in us. Everybody therefore is craving *feeling* something, to have a real *experience* of elevation. And they want it through community and shared experience. These are the natural desires of every human.

Get ready for a revolutionary truth—one that the billion-dollar drug and pharmaceutical industries do not want you to understand or practice—we can actually elevate ourselves and create the same chemicals in the brain that external substances open up. By using Kundalini Yoga, you actually activate the chemical distributions in the brain that are your *natural* chemical distributions. Because contrary to popular experience and therefore belief—our physical, mental, and emotional systems are totally wired to be happy and to feel good. We just have to access that wiring and activate it. This is the elementary premise behind Kundalini Yoga technology. The yoga is a form of practice that gives you immediate access to your fundamental and effervescent health and well-being.

This is why, unlike with a lot of other practices in the yoga world, you don't have to be crazy flexible to do Kundalini Yoga. You don't have to participate in the status quo physically obsessed yogic culture at all. In fact one of my favorite things is when people roll in to class straight from work or in between errands dressed in jeans or business clothes!

Kundalini Yoga is for men, women, moms, dads, students, busy professionals, artists, grandparents, kids, military vets, hospital patients, police officers, spiritual seekers, creatives . . . It's for everyone. Every body type, every health level, every phase of life. It always touches me when I have people in their seventies or eighties in the same room as teenagers, which is almost every class! It is for real people with real lives. The only barrier to entry is your desire to willingly participate in changing your life—which can be a big one!

The practices in the Kundalini Yoga teachings given by Yogi Bhajan over forty years of teaching in the West are the same ones you will find in this book, and they are easy enough for even the most out-of-shape individual yet still powerful enough to activate and expand even the most seasoned yogi or athlete. Luckily, if you find that you can't physically perform a certain breath practice, meditation, or exercise, I've also saturated this manual with lifestyle tips, dietary changes, and special yogic knowledge that will shift your whole being. If you want a change, even the smallest one, you have to change your movement patterns, your thought patterns, your eating patterns, your relating patterns—you have to change *something*! Even changing one little thing will make a significant shift in your daily experience.

DROP IN

In its true unadulterated essence, yoga is a powerful tool that you use for your own fulfillment *and* to hold a space on the planet for hope, potential, human goodness, and compassion. The physical practice is only a metaphor for the flexibility, power, and strength that develops in all parts of you as a whole being through these yogic practices. In the West, we have gotten fixated on the physical aspects of the practice, thinking that this is the sole reason to practice yoga of any sort.

In the 1960s hippie era, Timothy Leary popularized the counterculture phrase, "Turn on, tune in, drop out." This is a metaphor for why the revolution of the 1960s didn't come to fruition.

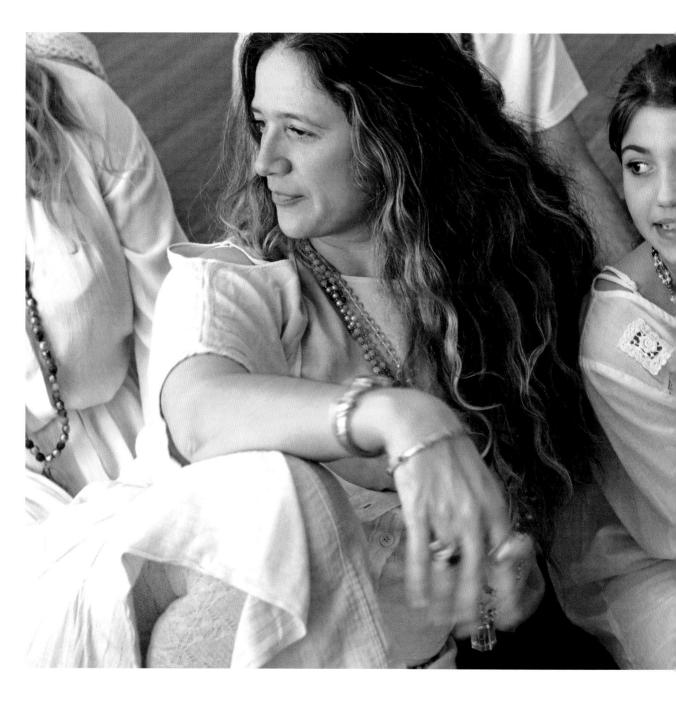

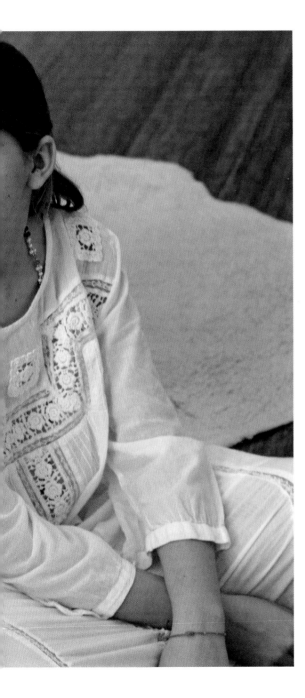

*Our practice has
the opportunity
to become a place
where we are so
engaged in our own
transformation
that we hold with
us a space for
hope, potential,
human goodness,
compassion,
and the energy
to become more
available to serve
others.*

The rallying cry of *this* age is only two letters different but represents the monumental shift happening as we speak: "Turn on, tune in, drop *in*!" The more we make space to turn toward our truest self, the more in rhythm we become with our mind, body, and therefore our experience of the external world or reality.

We have enough fear and terror on the planet right now. We want to and can elevate ourselves so that we can elevate each other. This is a New Revolution. It's now considered a revolutionary act to be happy in society today. A revolution is not necessarily going out on the streets to protest. New-era revolutionaries are those who have decided that they are going to be themselves, create for creation's sake, love themselves and others with abandon, and enjoy the precious life they have! From these fundamental decisions, a new way of creating and living in society is a natural outpouring of these elevated lifestyle choices.

Our practice has the opportunity to become a place where we are so engaged in our *own* transformation that we hold within us a space for hope, potential, human goodness, compassion, and the energy to become more available to serve others. To accomplish this, we must engage deeply in our own clarity and strengthening while simultaneously clearing the haze of self-centeredness that is so prolific in our culture today. Obsessing about what we look like and competing with ourselves and others—it's a very well-trodden path. But with each conscious breath, awareness literally comes to you in a flash and even greater change occurs on every level of your personal, professional, and creative life.

NOT YOUR AVERAGE NEW AGE

A lot of times, people don't want to do yoga because it seems very spiritual or physically demanding and they think they don't belong or don't buy into some pseudo-spiritual nonsense of it all. Kundalini Yoga *will* give you a spiritual experience—which I'll define here as an experience of the vastness of *you* in relationship to all there is—but it's not about spirituality and certainly not about the Institution of Spirituality, where the idea of being spiritual can become a very slippery slope and a caricature of itself very quickly.

Spirituality has too often been conflated with organized religion, which carries with it both negative and positive associations. Religion too often means that you belong to a certain faction of belief and that you follow whatever was written in a particular edited version of your belief system. There is a way to be good and a way to be bad, and if you aren't following the code for being a good religious person, you're doing it wrong. So oftentimes we drag a lot of our fears, hang-ups, and misunderstanding about religion into our spiritual pursuits, which are in truth simply desires for a deeper experience of ourselves, of God, of some Universal force, of our creativity, of love, of community, and of belonging to something bigger than ourselves.

Kundalini Yoga is a science. It's not about shamans and malas and incense—although everything can be used to discover a deeper part of yourself or create a Sacred Outlook on your world or your life. Using New Age tchotchkes and card decks as a replacement for your own authentic experience, however, starts to create the kind of stereotypical New Age fodder that has been such a turnoff to so many people. Tibetan Buddhist master and teacher Chögyam Trungpa Rinpoche aptly named this kind of spirituality Spiritual Materialism. In the old age of fluffy spirituality, there were a lot of New Agey teachers and people floating around spouting things like, "It's all about love and oneness." And it certainly is true—that's what it *is* all about. But using some spiritual know-how to glaze things over doesn't actually work to guide long-lasting changes in the patterns of neurons and thought waves that populate our neuroses or fear of the future. So this glazing-over type of spirituality or consumer spirituality is just another way we abort the mission of truly facing ourselves, having an authentic experience of being alive, and starting to generate and utilize enough energy in our body-mind system.

A truly "spiritual" moment is what happens when you're in the good, bad, and ugly of it all—*I'm angry right now . . . and I want to lash out at this guy . . . and he's called my husband*—and you have the wherewithal to do or think *something more creative, more expanded.* This requires a *how.* Kundalini Yoga provides you with an actionable and repeatable blueprint of how to achieve the things you want in your life through the countless and very simple *hows* of using your breath, your body, and your mind to direct and activate your own reality.

In the science of Kundalini Yoga, there is less interest in good and bad, and much more focus on the actual *experience.* The direct, powerful experience of you, your breath, and your life. How can you have a deeper experience of your own sensitivity or sensory system and then use that to have a deeper experience of whatever it is you want—love, prosperity, compassion, whatever? Kundalini Yoga allows you to become the creator of your own experience in concert with whatever creative forces you identify with, your personal experience, and your understanding of the generating, organizing, and developing or destroying forces of reality.

In the past, you most likely believed something because someone in religious or societal or familial power told you to believe it. In this new era, *you* decide if something resonates, and *you* decide if you want to take it on. When you have an experience, then that experience belongs to you. So I am sharing many of the most profound teachings and practices in Kundalini Yoga that can change your life in a powerful way, and I encourage you to pick up whatever works for you and practice it. Some of these practices are so simple, you could do them anywhere—no dim lighting, nag champa, or Buddha statue required.

However, wherever you are, you can maximize your practice if you tune in for a moment—even silently. The term *tuning in* refers to setting the space and also synchronizing your cellular and energetic system to a particular frequency. In Kundalini Yoga we do this with a sound code, *Ong Namo Guru Dev* (sounds like the *a* in *save*) *Namo.*

Sounds activate our brain, and these codes, also called mantras, activate our neurology in a certain way; the tongue and the teeth and how we move our lips activate all the quadrants of the brain. *Ong Namo Guru Dev Namo* essentially uplinks you to wisdom—yours and the collective—in order to guide your practice. When you use any kind of mantra or chanting, it is not necessarily the meaning of the sound but actually *the sound itself* that awakens these elevated levels of consciousness. So that's why we use the technology of sound to create a space for your practice.

When you find a practice that means something to you intuitively in this book, and you start to practice it because it just feels right, it's yours forever and the experience you cultivate cannot be taken away. And then you start to radiate with it. Then you start to vibrate with it. Then all sorts of things in your life begin to clear away and activate.

The practices of Kundalini Yoga are very much a process of biofeedback. When you practice Kundalini Yoga, it sends a signal, a command to the Universe. *I'm ready. I showed up this morning. I am showing up in my life. I'm engaging in a deeper resonance of my experience of being human. And I'm ready for more, and I'm ready for something that fits better with my current state of beingness and consciousness.* And since it's not new understanding that everything operates on vibrational resonance and frequency, you begin to generate a more heightened vibrational experience both internally and therefore externally.

In this book, you will find an ocean of deep, powerful, cosmic practices that will change your life. I've shifted my own experience in the most powerful ways—beyond what I could even explain in words—just using the technology of Kundalini Yoga. But of all the meditation and lifestyle tips and yogic secrets I have been taught and practice, from simple to wildly esoteric, one practice is the easiest and by far my favorite. So, as you take your first step in your new way of Invincible Living, I start you off with the accessible and powerful victory practice.

VICTORY

Nothing is more spiritual and, really, *braver* than waking up in the morning and summoning up the energy to face yourself, your life, and your tasks with solidarity, enjoyment, and vigilance! *That's* what spirituality is on a daily, momentary basis—making a conscious effort to replace your insecurities and self-doubt with the *victory* of your humanity. This is announcing that you've shown up on this planet, in your life, and that no matter what comes, you have enough energy and vitality to be with it in a way that will create growth and truth in not only you but also within anyone who comes into contact with you. This is the true *victory*!

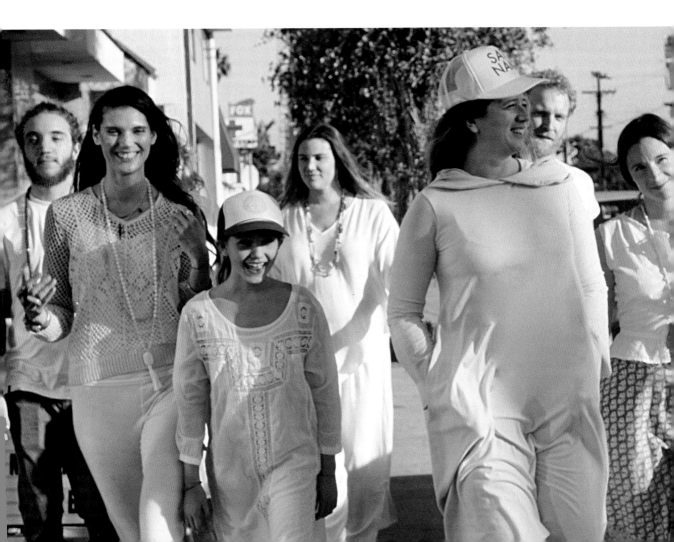

If you have the vitality, the energy to be victorious, you can ultimately touch your own spirit and the spirit of all that is. Victory. This is the mantra for this new time on the planet. That sound current—literally the word *victory* on your breath—will totally change your psychomagnetic frequency. When you put the sound *victory* on your own breath, then your whole psychomagnetic field broadcasts to the Universe a victorious experience and a victorious reality. So, with just one breath, you've already taken the leap from instability, insecurity, and the arrhythmia of your own neurosis to a place of fearlessness, security, personal awareness, and previously unimagined empowerment!

BREATH FOR VICTORY

NOTE: You can do this exercise no matter where you are, even if it's in line at the supermarket.

POSTURE: Sit or stand.

EYES: Keep your eyes closed, gently focusing up and in at the brow point.

BREATH AND MANTRA: Inhale and hold your breath. Press the tip of the tongue to the roof of the mouth. Mentally vibrate the mantra, *Victory!* Exhale. Repeat and continue. You can also hold the breath and mentally repeat, *Victory, victory, victory, victory* . . . as many times as you can in one breath. Exhale and repeat.

TIME: 10 seconds to 3 minutes

TO END: Inhale, exhale, and relax.

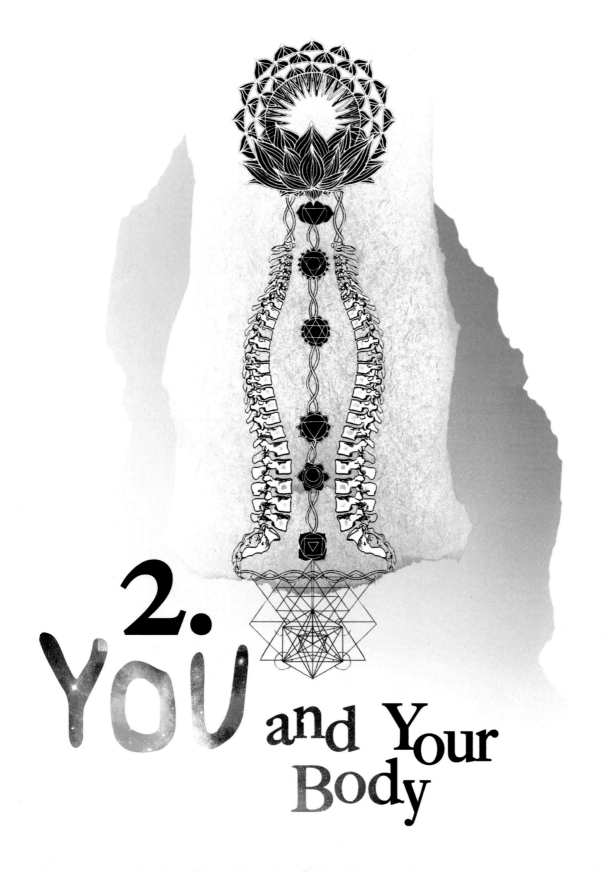

2.
YOU and Your Body

Your body gives you the power to move through life. When the body is strong, healthy, and resilient, life is enjoyable and exciting. When the body is sick, lacking energy, or just not reaching its radiant potential, life is challenging and frustrating.

Subtle, bio-intelligent adjustments make all the difference in rejuvenating and regenerating your body. You don't need to blow through your savings on a spa weekend or spend half your paycheck on premium supplements. When you understand the sophisticated systems of your body, you can tune these systems for health, radiance, and vibrancy—for *free*. It just takes a little time and effort, like anything that's good in life. The key is knowing what parts of your body govern your vitality and how to adjust them. You can actually set the vibrancy of your longevity for the next twenty years of your life with just one of the Kundalini Yoga practices in this book, giving you youthfulness, a healthy lifespan, and extended vitality.

But, just as financial advisers tell you to start saving for retirement at thirty, the earlier you can begin to adjust, replenish, and refuel your body systems, the longer they will last. And of course, no matter how old you are, you can always make a massive impact on your daily and long-term health experience through these practices.

We all want tools that open up, rejuvenate, and activate a happy, healthy physical body. This technology has those tools. However, we also all have some resistance to unrolling the mat—or sheepskin, in Kundalini Yoga—and getting to work.

Some of that is just mind resistance. You're tired. You can't do the poses. You don't know what kind of yoga set to do. You don't want to get ready and get out of the house to go somewhere for class. You'll do it tomorrow when you have more time.

But there's also that resistance to yoga because it's, well, too much like *yoga*. Even I have to admit there's sometimes nothing more obnoxious than some twenty-two-year-old, two-hundred-hour-trained yoga teacher spouting Sanskrit names about different parts of your body that you don't know, can't do, or just plain don't understand.

But part of what all yoga offers is its sophistication. Because your physical system is elaborately unique and specialized, yoga has to be aware of your body's complex and differentiated systems, which sometimes, though not always, requires fancy esoteric names. Developed from more than five thousand years of physioenergetic experimentation, yoga in all of its forms is powerful yet refined practices that awaken, activate, heal, and amplify your total body. And not just the physical body; in Kundalini Yoga we become aware of and exercise our whole *ten-body* system.

YOUR TEN-BODY SYSTEM

In reality, your physical body is only one-tenth of your total embodied experience. In a lot of spiritual systems, you'll see the breakdown of embodiment into three planes of experience (mind-body-spirit). Still others break it down into five or seven planes of total sensitivity. The sophisticated yogis of *this* lineage identified ten bodies of experience. Cleanliness, functionality, and utilization on all ten levels creates the most vitalized feeling of living and the most creative, intelligent navigation of the life landscape.

Your ten bodies include:

1. **SOUL BODY:** The indivisible vibration that is *you* beyond time and space.

2. **NEGATIVE MIND:** That which sees possible pitfalls and potholes in the road ahead—protective.

3. **POSITIVE MIND:** That which sees all the opportunities available to you in any given moment—supportive.

4. **NEUTRAL MIND:** That which synthesizes all data from the negative and positive minds and gives a directive of action or inaction based on the needs of the soul—your true *you.*

5. **PHYSICAL BODY:** That which we know as the physiological, biological beingness.

6. **ARCLINE:** The baseline auric structure that holds incarnational patterns and blessings. It runs from earlobe to earlobe in both men and women. A second arcline extends from nipple to nipple in women only.

7. **AURA:** The combined energetic field of your chakras, which are wheels of energy generated by dense crosshairs of nerve fibers and biochemicals, and which have actual location in the physical body.

8. **PRANIC BODY:** That which holds your life force in the physical form. It is regulated by the breath.

9. **SUBTLE BODY:** Also known as the ghost's body. When your physical body perishes, the subtle body and the soul body join together and travel to the next stage of being—whatever that is. The subtle body is attenuated, deeply artistic, and profound.

10. RADIANT BODY: The body that glorifies you, allows you to project into the world, and attracts success and also dispels negativity and darkness wherever you go.

When all ten bodies are running high, connecting to each other, and operating under your conscious control and relationship, this gives you an eleventh body—the embodiment—the integration into unison—unified by the harmonics and vibrations of Sound itself.

This ten-body experience can be really energizing and intuitive, but if it's coming off as a little too esoteric, skip ahead to something you can bite your teeth into. We don't want to get caught up in fancy yogic terms for the sake of some idea and lose sight of the point of yogic technology—which is just to *feel better* now and into the future.

The point of yoga is to give you a better experience of life. If something resonates with you and you can apply one or more of these bodies to make more creative, intelligent decisions in your *life,* then great. But if not, keep it simple and direct. The whole point of knowing that these bodies exist and how they function is so that you can improve your real life and empower your existence. And maybe—just maybe—feel a little less imprisoned and fixated on just your physical experience, although it *is* intrinsically important to create a baseline for your life.

The thing that really sets Kundalini Yoga apart from other forms of yoga is that every yoga set, meditation, or technique heals and amplifies all ten bodies at the same time. If you're working out, you may tone up your *physical* body, but that's one-tenth of the whole deal! That's why it's not uncommon to see highly fitness-focused people not actually looking or feeling that well or healthy. Something needs to be balanced in their *whole* system.

It's one thing to be flexible in your body, like something you could achieve with a regular yoga class. In Kundalini Yoga technology, the basis of the technology is that it creates agility in *all* areas of your life, all of your bodies. You have nine other bodies that you need to be agile in order for you

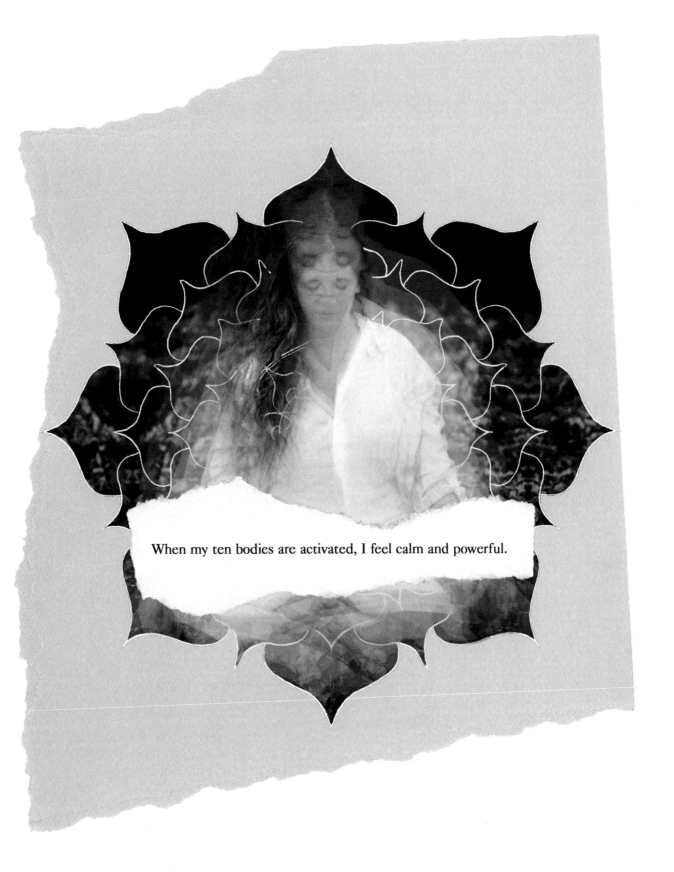

When my ten bodies are activated, I feel calm and powerful.

to be able to maneuver through time in space in a way that has grace. And frankly, the world is in need of more grace, and people who are interested in being graceful in the way they treat themselves, each other, and the planet.

To get in touch with your ten-body system, the best practice is to do a full yoga set, or *kriya*. In the center of the book, "Invincible Living Tips," you will find some of my favorite yoga sets. You can discover the one that best suits you and practice it daily, or you can do a new one each day.

In the meantime, remember that a healthy body gives you the flexibility, strength, and sensory refinement to move through life with security, stability, grace, inspiration, and majesty. It simply feels better to have a body that works well at any age. This is why I want you to focus here on your physical body, that which we know as our physiological, biological vehicle, which is vastly sacred and beautiful.

PHYSICAL WISDOM

Your physical body is a vibrant masterpiece of different physical systems. It's like a piece of art, with many layers and many colors. When studying anatomy, I personally feel closer to some deeper meaning than at any other time. God, Universe, whatever you want you call it, something deeper, something elemental. This physical system is *just so beautiful, perfect, and poetic*. The top systems that have the biggest impact on how you experience life are:

THE MUSCULOSKELETAL SYSTEM

THE GLANDULAR SYSTEM

THE ORGANS OF THE BODY

THE NERVOUS SYSTEM

THE METABOLIC SYSTEM

We could go so in depth into human anatomy in a 101 kind of way. But I'd like to show you how each system in your body creates your spectrum of emotions, thoughts, and experiences—your version of reality. When your body starts to change, your reality changes. Just a cubic centimeter more of lung capacity changes your whole outlook on life—it expands you! So I think it's important to note not just how these systems work but also how they instruct and format your life view.

THE MUSCULOSKELETAL SYSTEM

As the primary framework of your body, the musculoskeletal system is the main determinant to how tall you are, your stature, your strength, your carriage, the qualities of your movement, and the geometry of your being. The muscles and the bones of your body work together to mobilize you and hold the experience of *being* in a body.

Yoga can do a lot to heal this foundational physical structure. For instance, something as simple as deep, yogic breathing increases bone strength and density by creating more minerals in the body and delivering them deep into your bone marrow. Yogic poses and exercises stretch, tone, and strengthen the muscles in the body.

By far the most important part of the musculoskeletal system is your *spinal column*. Your spinal column is an elegant and massively important chain of vertebrae that affects and controls almost every other aspect of the body. The spine houses the central nervous system, which in turn commands your peripheral nervous system, which in turn regulates and directs all the muscles in the body, the organs, the glands, and even the brain. A healthy, flexible spinal column *directly* translates to a healthy nervous system, which in turn regulates the rest of the bodily functions in a balanced, enjoyable way.

Every yogic tradition has some version of the same saying, "Youth is in

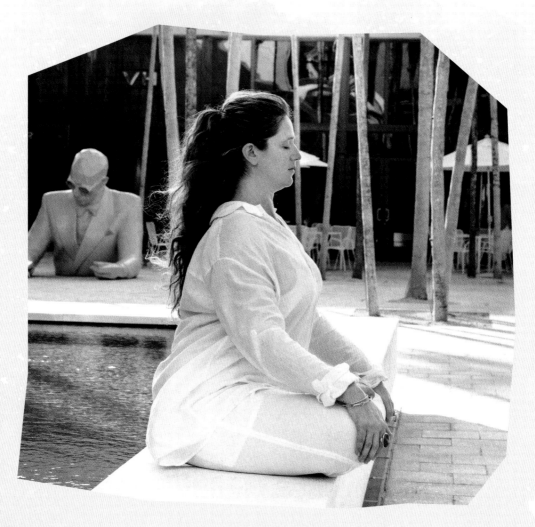

CAMEL FLEX

POSTURE: Sit in a cross-legged position, a.k.a. easy pose. Grab your shins with both hands.

EYES: Keep your eyes closed, gently focusing up and in at the brow point.

BREATH: Inhale. Flex the spine forward and open your chest. Then exhale, flex the spine backward and, without collapsing your chest, stretch your lower spine. Try to keep your head level—don't swing your chin up and down as you flex; move just your spine.

TIME: 1 to 3 minutes

TO END: Inhale and bring your spine back to a neutral position. Then stretch your body and spine up. Exhale and relax.

the flexibility of the spine." When the spinal column has flexion and mobility, you feel healthy, happy, and vitalized. But when the spine is stiff, out of alignment, or somehow dislocated, it doesn't matter if you're fifteen years old or sixty years old; you'll feel like you're eighty-five.

With consistent yogic practice, spinal health can actually be restored quite easily. Even if you've had long-standing back issues, like a slipped or compressed disk, you can realign yourself quickly and even add fullness and cushion to your aging disks. One of my favorite exercises for spinal health is called the Camel Flex. The exercise is simple but profoundly effective.

THE GLANDULAR SYSTEM

The glandular system is sometimes also referred to as the endocrine system. It affects your emotions, your aging process, your immunity, your metabolism, *and* your general sense of wellness. Your ability to handle stresses and challenges, even the smallest things in life, is directly related to your glandular system functioning. When you experience the joy and thrills of life, that's *also* your glandular system reacting to them. Your glands work together with the nervous system to give you "experiences," which are ultimately—whether we like it or not—what we have come to experience in a human body, no matter how challenging or uncomfortable!

Many other chapters in this book cover the nuances of the glandular system as it relates to a specific facet of life. But if I can give you one quick takeaway here that will change your life, it's that the glands are the keepers of youth, health, and beauty. Care for them and you will have a more immediate and long-term experience of immaculate health and vitality.

One of the easiest ways to care for your glandular system is with balanced eating. Undereating or overeating of any kind really taxes the organs and the glands, particularly after you turn thirty-six (or even over eighteen). Taxing your organs and glands leads to accelerated aging. It's one of the reasons that

BREATH OF FIRE

POSTURE: Sit in easy pose with your hands resting on your knees in gyan mudra (with the tips of your index finger and thumb touching).

EYES: Keep your eyes closed, gently focusing up and in at the brow point.

BREATH: Begin an even inhale and even exhale through the nose. The breath should be strong and rapid, but *even*. Do not overemphasize the exhale or put too much emphasis on the navel point. Even inhale, even exhale.

TIME: 3 to 11 minutes

TO END: Inhale deeply, stretch your body up, exhale, and relax.

I'm against extended juice cleansing for most people, especially women. I give some more directives about food later on, but for now, in the culture that praises self-starvation and late-night binges on fast food, it's important to just remember that balance is key.

If you've had a history of extremes in dieting, or if you've had kids or have been on birth control for any amount of time, or if your doctor has mentioned a hormonal imbalance, there are potent yogic tools to reset your glands quickly and effectively! One of the basic exercises that will get your glandular system (and hormones) in order is Breath of Fire for seven minutes a day. When you hit that seven-minute mark, the pituitary and pineal glands start to release a very specific secretion that puts the glands back into balance. The pituitary

Activate your radiant body!

BREATH

OF FIRE

COLD SHOWER

DIRECTIONS:

1. Dry brush your body in short strokes toward the heart from the base of your feet all the way up. The skin should become pink. If you dry brush the skin of your face, which you can, do so gently and stroke upward.

2. Massage almond oil or coconut oil all over your body, including your face.

3. Turn on the cold water in your shower and get in.

4. Facing the water, begin massaging different parts of your body, starting with the soles of your feet and continuing with the tops of your feet and your hands.

5. To treat the back of the body, turn around and let the cold water run down your spine. Rub your shoulders, armpits, upper arms, forearms, and wrists on both sides. Rub your kidneys and lower back. Strike the buttocks lightly. Massage the back of your calves with the tops of your feet, and then turn around again.

6. Massage your face. Let the water hit your chest and massage your heart center and breasts. Massage your stomach. Then lightly strike the tops of your thighs with loose fists.

TIME: 30 seconds to 15 minutes, or until you are warm

TO END: Get out of the shower; towel yourself off till you are totally dry. Look in the mirror, admire your glow!

gland controls all other glandular secretions, so if you balance that, you can balance the whole body.

By far, one of my all-time favorite practices for glandular health *and* overall youth and rejuvenation is the Cold Shower.

This practice is an incredible kind of hydrotherapy. It improves the integrity and condition of the skin. It detoxes the inner organs, increases immunity, fends off depression, heals the circulatory system, erases wrinkles, activates cellular renewal, improves energy, strengthens the nerves, and even makes your brain more alert by increasing the velocity of your neurons. Cold showers are the best bet for fast glandular reset—and, as an added bonus, they make you feel incredible.

I know what you're thinking . . . *Eff no!* But I promise you, this is one of the most amazing, fast-acting, antiaging, rejuvenating practices you could ever take on. The oil application described opposite really offsets the shock of the cold water and deeply moisturizes your skin. It's a quickie version of an ancient Ayurvedic practice called Abhiyanga, the external application of oil to nourish your organs.

THE ORGANS OF THE BODY

The organ system covers a broad range of your inner anatomy. Bodily organs include everything from the skin to the stomach to the lungs to the ovaries. For our purposes, I'm considering any kind of tissue in the body with a specific function a part of this system.

The important thing to know about organs is that they *work*. They have jobs, like digesting your food or metabolizing oxygen. And because they work, they can get taxed, exhausted, and backed up if not cared for properly.

Most of us are dealing with some kind of organ fatigue in the body on some level. Every day your organs literally process airfreights of food and toxicity from air pollution, weird foods, stress, synthetic cosmetics, and much more. When your organs don't get the nourishment they need, they overwork and fall into fatigue or failure. If you feel as if you don't have the stamina to do simple things, like return that phone call or get yourself ready for work, you are most likely dealing with a level of organ toxicity or fatigue.

The funny thing about organ fatigue is that no amount of time you spend on vacation in Hawaii will heal your organs unless you use some direct yogic or detoxing practice to deeply cleanse and rejuvenate. Everyone wants to take an exit from "normal life." But you can still feel sick and fatigued in Kauai, and a lot of people do!

Your organs need to be cleansed and supported. They process so much for the body that incremental bits of unprocessed waste start to add up until the organs are totally overstressed and, most likely, toxic. Lethargy, adult acne, weight gain, aging, joint pain, and lack of flexibility are all results of organ toxicity.

Cold showers are phenomenal for detoxing the organs, as is one of my favorite techniques of fasting on specific Lunar Days!

The New Moon, the Fourth Day of the Moon, the Eleventh Day of the Moon, and the Full Moon are powerful days for organ detox. On these days, the unique phase of the moon pulls on the waters in the body in a highly specific way. The result of is a very subtle, bio-celestial interaction that naturally triggers the body into self-healing and internal repair. Juice fasting or liquid dieting on these four lunar phases amplifies the curative effects of the day and deeply nourishes the whole body.

For me, this also takes the place of extended juice detoxes. Four single-day fasts per lunar cycle ends up being fifty-two days of fasting a year! Which has been a huge boost to my metabolic and digestive efficiency without hurting the body.

In addition to detoxing, your organs need to be massaged and conditioned. Healthy glandular secretion will condition your organs with a healing internal serum, keeping them young and functional. And yogic poses that involve compression, stretching, or heavy breathing will also detox and massage

MASTER SET NO. 1

1. Come sitting in baby pose, sitting on your heels, arms by your side, forehead toward or on the ground and palms facing up. Keep your chest on your thighs. Lift only your head off the ground, and begin a Breath of Fire. Continue for 1½ to 3 minutes.

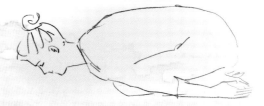

2. Staying on your heels, if possible, or coming to easy crossed-legged pose, slowly roll down and lie down onto your back. Open up the front part of your body, and begin another Breath of Fire. Continue for 1½ to 3 minutes.

3. Come slowly out of the posture and into a squat variation. Bring your legs out wide and squat so that your thighs are parallel to the ground. Take your arms inside of the legs, and then grasp your heels or top of feet from the inside. Come onto your toes if you need to or keep feet on ground more preferably. Lift your torso as much as you can. Stick your tongue out of your mouth, and begin a Breath of Fire through the mouth. Continue 1½ to 3 minutes.

4. Inhale, exhale, and relax.

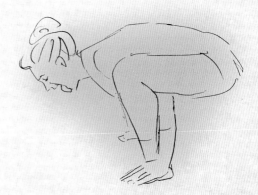

the organs for revitalized internal health. One of my favorite yoga exercises for internal massage and conditioning of the organs and glands is called the Master Set No. 1.

THE NERVOUS SYSTEM

Your nervous system is a vast, sophisticated system of internal wiring and biochemical carriers that communicate life experiences. This amazing feat of biological evolution plays an immense role in our relation to the world and also how we navigate it. The nervous system literally relates situations from the outside world to the glands for hormonal release, the total of which we call experience. It also sends signals to the brain and the muscles about what to do next, how to navigate our lives.

You actually have three parts to your nervous system: the central nervous system, the sympathetic nervous system, and the parasympathetic nervous system. I go into more depth on these parts of the nervous system in chapter 5—"Fully Stress-Free." But I think what's most crucial to understand about this part of the body is that it runs on electricity, which means it conducts *wattage*.

Just like you can't run 200 volts of electricity through a 20-watt cable without frying the wires, if your nervous system isn't primed and strong, you can't handle huge stress waves—or huge joy waves!—without your system totally shutting down. That's why so many more people than ever before are experiencing mental, emotional, and physical breakdowns. We all have high-stress jobs and live in high-stress environments. No matter where you live or what you do for a living or your financial and familial responsibilities, you have stress and challenges between you and your dreams. If your nervous system hasn't been tempered and fortified, you will experience this short-circuiting.

And the level of wattage your nervous system can conduct is equal to the amount of happiness you can experience. You can't run huge prosperity waves—which are just more energy showing up as money, promotions, and expansions of all kinds—through your system if it can't handle the voltage. You can't run huge waves of love through your system either. Love, happiness, and wealth require strength to hold and enjoy. Love and light are *real,* but if you don't have the nervous system strength to actually conduct that experience, it's just another New Age cliché.

Nervous system failure is also part of the whole violence situation on the planet right now. More and more often we hear stories on the news about increases in police violence and gun violence in general. This is in part due to weakened nervous systems in the population as well as problems with shortness of breath, lack of exercise, poor nutrition, excessive use of prescription and over-the-counter drugs that weaken the central nervous system and change brain chemistry, and many other factors of modern living. This is why nervous system health is one of the biggest things we have to take care of on an individual and societal basis.

Eating alkaline foods, taking cold showers (of course), and meditating will all help strengthen your nervous system. I'm also a big proponent of *hydration*! I know this seems all too basic, but you have no idea how many people are walking around dehydrated without even realizing it.

You need to be drinking half your body weight in ounces of water or fresh juice every day or at least trying to get close to it. You'd be amazed at how much more normal, relaxed, and happy you feel in a well-hydrated body. Also, good fats help the body to feel hydrated. These include middle-chain fatty acids like coconut oil, DHA, essential fatty acid blends, ghee, and avocado. Anytime you get stressed or worked up, just drink a full glass of water, breathe, and then act. Watch how it changes the way you respond to ordinarily stressful situations.

THE METABOLIC SYSTEM

The metabolic system is how the body processes and utilizes energy. For yogic purposes, we'll say this is *any* kind of energy, from *prana* (life force energy available anywhere but most easily accessed through breath) to caloric energy of food. There are many kinds of metabolic activities going on in your system at any given time, but the kind that we are most familiar with is the digestive metabolism.

Yogic teachings around food are a huge topic, partly because one of the positive trends of the wellness industry is that we are becoming more aware of output and input on all levels. In yogic tech this includes what we say, what we eat, how we breathe, how we receive love—the list goes on and on. But food is very important to talk about. Even though we want to gain an awareness and sensitivity to more subtle forms of processing energy, we also want to start with something we can actually make changes in right away. And digestive metabolism is easy, obvious, and highly impactful on how you enjoy your body and experience your day. So this is a very good place to start.

One of my missions as a yogi in the modern age is to find new ways to relate with our body and food, to basically pave a way for a whole new experience for ourselves and those who come after us. There is so much neurosis around our fixation with our physical body, and yet the proper care and usage of the physical body is so rewarding!

You're metabolizing a lot of energy on a daily basis in the modern speed of a life, and all that energy gets sent through the nervous system. And we know that when you send that much energy though the nervous system and your nervous system hasn't been primed, you're setting yourself up for eventual breakdown. That's why an overactive metabolism might mean you burn off weight, maybe, but can create an overactive mind and emotions.

On the flip side, an underactive metabolism leaves you feeling slug-

LUNAR CYCLE

I use the cycle of the moon for my greatest health. On the four lunar days, our bodies naturally renew themselves. I fast and/or eat greens during these times to support rejuvenation and antiaging.

gish. Depressed. Fatigued. And overweight, which means you are carrying excess physical and emotional baggage that you don't want. If you have a sluggish metabolism and a hard time losing weight, raising your metabolic rate is something you'll want to work on. But it's important to know that a *high* metabolism isn't always a healthy metabolism or even an *enjoyable* one.

It's super trendy right now to go on a weeklong juice cleanse. But if you're over thirty, extended fasts and juice cleanses are not necessarily recommended, and they won't really deliver the results you're looking for in a long-lasting way. This is due in part to the metabolic slowing that happens when you shut down your digestion. After three days, your body may start to store fat rather than shed it because the body goes into starvation response. Again, this is more prevalent in women over thirty, as our bodies have a big hormonal and endocrine shift at that time.

As I mentioned, I recommend fasting for a day at a time on specific lunar days (new moon, fourth day of the moon, eleventh day of the moon, and the full moon). Fasting on these days helps support the new secretions, and you start to feel friendlier, more patient, and more compassionate while your body starts to come into its highest beauty. You may notice that your personality actually changes when your endocrine functioning changes and your metabolism changes—it's perceptible. This is important because a healthy glandular system in humans is deeply connected to the new era of society that we're building—one in which we are naturally happy, healthy, and therefore kinder to ourselves and others.

If you are looking for an extended metabolic reboot, I am an advocate of *mono diets*. Mono diets are food plans where you eat only one kind of food, or one kind of meal, for a set period of time. Yogi Bhajan assigned and taught many, many types of mono diets for different reasons. Eating steamed beets and their greens exclusively for three days or eating only watermelon for a week are healthy examples of mono dieting. You can do mono diets for weeks, in some cases even months, to help you lose weight,

Whenever I'm feeling lackluster, I go on three days of the Green Diet. It completely brightens the skin, lifts mood, and delivers activated energy! It seems restrictive, but actually green foods exist in abundance. Some of my favorites include:

The Green Diet

* Green apples
* Pears
* Grapes
* Honeydew melon
* Wheatgrass
* Avocado
* Nori
* Pistachios
* Pumpkin seeds
* Olives and olive oil
* Hemp seeds
* Hemp milk
* Kale, spinach, and all leafy green lettuces
* Broccoli
* Artichoke
* Asparagus
* Okra
* Snap peas
* Green beans
* more . . .

To add a little variety to this mono diet, you can season your meals with any organic spice, organic soy or tamari sauce, or liquid aminos. Remember, any food is on this cleanse provided that it's organic, unprocessed, and naturally green!

heal your organs, reset your glands, improve your condition, and feel great about your body.

The benefit of a mono diet is that it gives the digestive system and organ system a break while keeping the *fiber* going. This is really crucial because the fiber is what keeps the metabolism going, the *Agni* (digestive fire) going, so that you actually continue to lose weight and detoxify. You get the benefit of the detoxification in a very simple way without taxing your organs with lack of nourishment or even suppressing your metabolism by restricting the number of calories and nutrients it can burn. With extended juice fasting, your metabolism can go into hibernation. So almost always, the moment you start eating again, you gain more weight than you lost.

So I really love these mono diets. And the bonus is that yogis have been doing them for thousands of years, so we know they work!

Some of my favorite mono diets include:

ONE WEEK OF STEAMED BEETS AND THEIR GREENS (OLIVE OIL OR COCONUT OIL AND SEASONINGS ALLOWED): This cleanse is good for liver stagnation. It heals the skin, especially acne issues, takes care of weight fluctuations, abates caffeine addiction, and eases any kind of habitual irritability or anger.

THREE TO FORTY DAYS OF ONLY GREEN FOODS: This mono diet reduces inflammation in the body, brightens you, makes you feel amazing, and is a great prenatal cleanse! The best part about the green diet is that it's actually very moderate, inexpensive, and easy. The key to the green diet is that it has to be any *naturally* green food and preferably organic. I have a really sweet student who, in the early days of Kundalini Yoga, thought that a green diet meant she could eat green M&M's and she literally used to pick them out of the bag just to eat!

ONE WEEK OF STEAMED TURNIPS MASHED WITH ALMOND OIL (OR COCONUT OIL), TURMERIC, LEMON, AND PEPPER: This mono diet heals the metabolism and the digestive system. It is also a great way to do a total organ detox while still feeling like you're getting to eat something really rich and delicious.

THREE TO FORTY DAYS OF MUNG BEANS AND RICE CALLED KITCHARI: This is a classic yogi mono diet. Major nerve renewal comes from this cleanse. It's healing and grounding. It restores the intestines and rebuilds all the tissues in the body.

3 · Endless BEAUTY

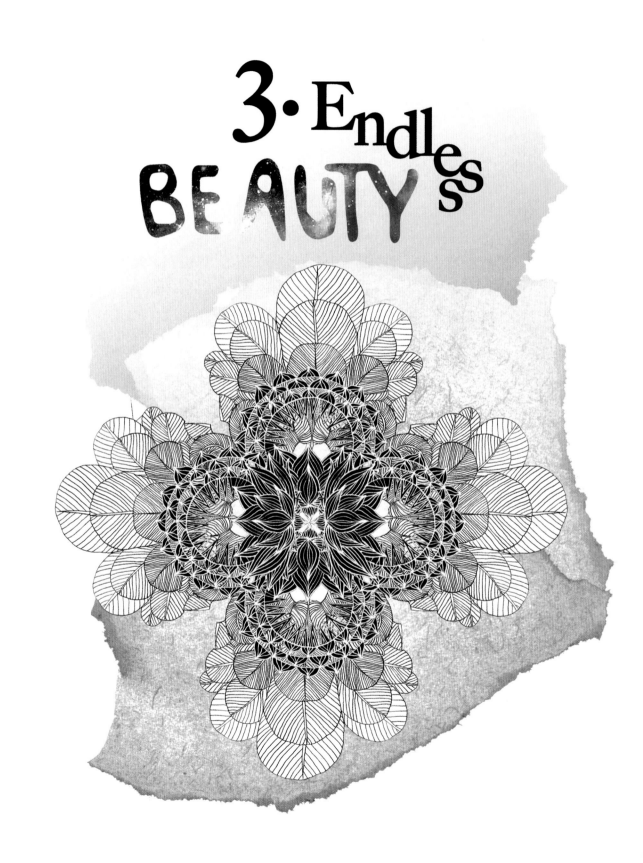

For *millennia,* women and men have been indoctrinated into fixed ideas about what aging and beauty look like. As a yogi you have the power to create a graceful, high-functioning aging process. The physical body is ultimately a finite machine, one that will one day wear out and die. But this doesn't mean that radiant, magnetic, and long-lasting inner and outer beauty *isn't* achievable. It is. The techniques to achieve this kind of endless beauty go far beyond food trends, premium topicals, or even the cultivation of an inner beauty.

Welcome to the next level of beauty consciousness. Kundalini Yoga gives you a naturally radiant, balanced, and vital physical experience and appearance.

It's due time to break through our deep societal media-driven conditioning around beauty and aging. In *reality,* with the right techniques, you can stay vital, vibrant, and luminous for as long as you want.

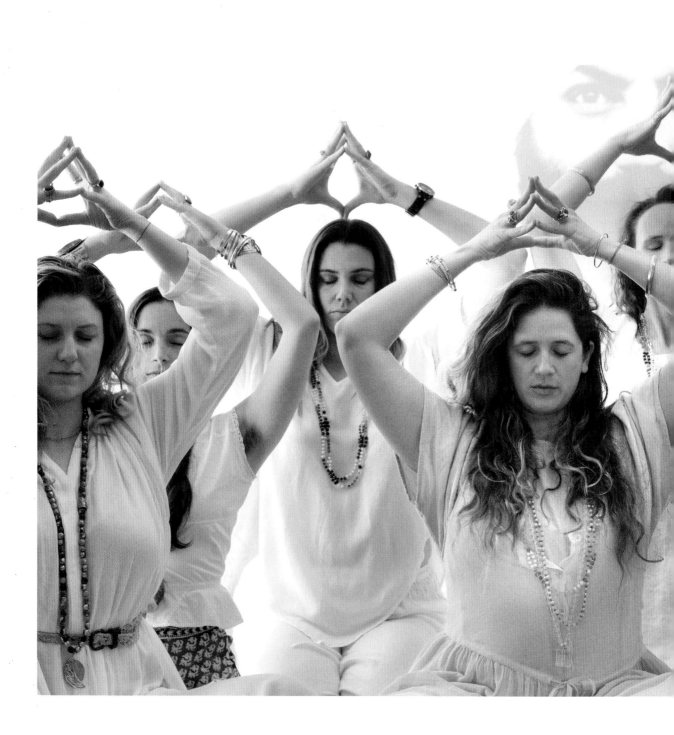

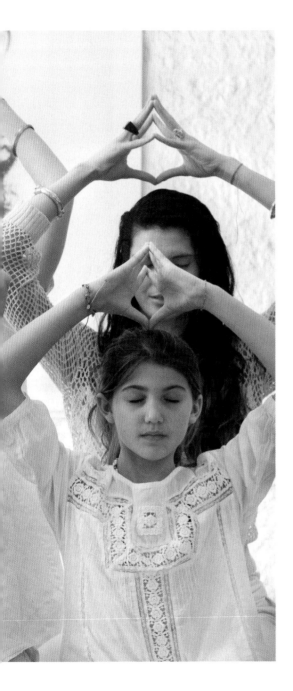

You must learn to look beyond the mirror. You are the spirit. You are the self. You are the honor. You are the source of all sources. You are redeemer of all redeemers. From you this creation is born.

—YOGI BHAJAN

BREAKING OUT OF DEEP CONDITIONING

The media broadcasts messages about beauty and youth that are intensely powerful and hypnotic. For example, do you feel like you need to "lose those last ten pounds"? This is one of those thought forms that affects millions of woman particularly, even though it literally has nothing to do with them or the state of their bodies and health. You can look incredible, be in the best shape of your life, and still be affected by the notion of the "last ten pounds." The idea is endemic and completely created by the media.

It's exciting that more and more people in Hollywood and the fashion industry, where much of this propaganda is generated, are starting to speak out about the ridiculousness of the double standards for women in our society. And more role models of different shapes and sizes are indicative of this consciousness shift. It takes a lot of strength and bravery for anyone, but especially women, to feel alive and embodied in their own skin no matter what their size, age, and shape. And the reality is that there is a heavy fear of aging in our collective consciousness that we all, men and women, have to deal with. Men have other aspects of the pressure of aging that are maybe more subtle but just as heavy in some ways.

There is a true opportunity now for all of us to create new personal relationships with aging and, ultimately, with dying. How we relate to the passing of time and space. How we relate to wisdom and the elders in society. All of these things are connected.

I've been through the gamut of health and spiritual practice. I spent time as a nutritional consultant, a cleanse expert, a Hatha yogi, and with many master teachers and yogis. In my vast experience, I've found that the most effective tools for breaking out of the negative beauty trance are in Kundalini Yoga. With immense methods for mind, health, and radiance, there is no faster, more effective system on the planet today.

These practices not only will help you personally to feel more vibrant and combat aging and disease on multiple levels, but they will also help us create a

YOGIC PRACTICE TO BREAK THE MEDIA SPELL AND ACTIVATE BEAUTY

Yogi Bhajan, the great yogi who brought Kundalini Yoga to the West, gave this powerful practice for breaking through old programming and replacing those thoughts with a new total beauty experience.

DIRECTIONS: Stand naked in front of a full-length mirror. Looking at yourself, repeat the mantra, *I am bountiful, blissful, and beautiful. Bountiful, blissful, and beautiful am I.* Continue to look at yourself and repeat the mantra for 1 to 11 minutes. To end, inhale, close your eyes, and feel your vastness.

world that is more courageous around difference, around wisdom, and around life and death. The following practices work to create a biochemistry of compassion for ourselves and others. The effects are astounding and cumulative, even more powerful than we may ever see or know.

THE REALITY OF PERPETUAL YOUTH

Because of the seriously calcified ideas we've adopted around aging, it bears repeating: You do *not* have to get wrinkles. You do *not* have to lose vitality, gain weight, or lose tone, mind clarity, energy, or the glow of youth. You do *not* have to age in the way we've been taught!

For *aeons*, yogic practice has produced a plentitude of individuals called *baal yogis*. Baal yogis are men and women who appear eternally youthful, as though suspended in time in a seemingly ageless state. One of these yogis was a man named Baba Siri Chand. Baba Siri Chand is one of the most powerful yogis of the Kundalini Yoga lineage, and it is said that in his *documented* 150 years of life, he looked forever like a boy. And Baba Siri Chand is just one of many yogis who have achieved such a feat.

To stop age in its tracks, it would take a level of yogic enlightenment heretofore unknown in the West. So I'm really not suggesting you go for baal yogi status, although you never know what can happen one day in meditation! What I think these powerful yogic cases show us is that we really don't have to go through the whole loss of skin tone, fine lines, deep wrinkles, thinning hair, graying and aging process the way we've been told! Techniques to turn back the clock and rejuvenate your glow do exist and we can utilize them today!

One of my all-time favorite glandular-resetting exercises is the Cat-Cow. I love Cat-Cow because it's so easy. You can do it almost anywhere, it doesn't require any special yogic ability, and it's colossally powerful!

Almost no one knows about the massively antiaging benefits of Cat-Cow. Just three to five minutes a day completely resets the glandular system, rebuilds body tissue, and totally rejuvenates your system. Cat-Cow is vitalizing, energizing and even builds collagen production in the face. In Kundalini Yoga, we call Cat-Cow a complete exercise, or kriya, because it also tunes your chakras and enhances your ten-body system. So if you could add just one exercise to your repertoire, I highly recommend the Cat-Cow at a good pace with deep breath.

YOGIC BEAUTY SECRETS

The real secret of your long-lasting inner and outer beauty is in your *glands*.

Glands produce hormones and special internal conditioning serums. When the glands secrete the correct rate for your body, it's like a balm or a lotion for your entire system. Your skin becomes firm, luscious, and conditioned. Your hair thickens and develops a glossy sheen. Your teeth and gums radiate cleanliness that's beyond oral care. Your eyes start to shine. Even your body odor starts to emanate as a natural freshness.

Yogis know that the glands are the keepers of your health, youth, and beauty, and over the millennia, yoga has produced the most effective methods for glandular adjustment. What always blows my mind about Kundalini Yoga is that some of these practices are *so easy* and *so effective*. For instance, you can stretch your elbows two or three times per day to keep your glandular system in tune. When practiced daily for forty days, this simple exercise will deliver a significant return of glow to your face!

LEFT-NOSTRIL BREATHING FOR HEALTHY EATING

NOTES: This exercise is also called Restraining Compulsive Eating. You can do it wherever you are, even if you can't get into easy pose. Breaths should be deep, but not exaggerated. Relaxed breathing, relaxed mind. Heal yourself.

POSTURE: Sit in easy pose.

EYES: Keep your eyes closed, gently focusing up and in at the brow point.

BREATH: Close your right nostril with your right thumb. Inhale deeply through your left nostril and hold your breath to capacity. Exhale your breath through the left nostril and hold your breath out for the same amount of time.

TIME: 3 to 11 minutes, or as needed

TO END: Inhale, exhale, and relax.

CAT-COW

POSTURE: Position yourself on your hands and knees.

EYES: Keep your eyes closed, gently focusing up and in at the brow point.

BREATH: Inhale as you stretch your chest open and lift your head, moving into cow pose. Exhale as you curl your back and pull your navel in toward your spine, cat pose. Repeat, continuing at a moderate pace and increasing the speed and power of your breath as you gain flexibility of the spine. Do not be afraid to breathe deeply and move quickly! The more quickly you move, the more antiaging benefits you receive!

TIME: 3 to 5 minutes

TO END: Inhale and stretch the body up into cow. Exhale and pull the navel in. Inhale to a neutral spine and relax the buttocks to your heels, bringing your forehead to the ground, stretching your arms on the floor in front of you, and placing your hands together.

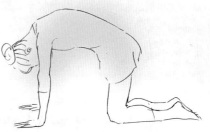

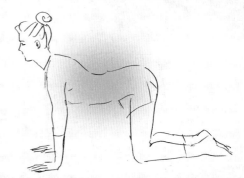

You can also simply eliminate your sugar intake. I always tell the women and men who come to my classes to watch how deeply they are addicted to sugar. Sugar is in everything these days, and Yogi Bhajan called it "very polite" how it enters your diet, and that it is *the enemy of youth*." To restore your vibrant glow, it can be as easy as minimizing sugar of any kind in your diet. This includes agave and brown sugar. Raw honey in small doses can be very medicinal, as well as stevia, an herb that has all sorts of health properties but also naturally sweetens.

A tendency to overeat or stress eat (and who doesn't have this?) also throws the glandular system off. It's important not to get into any kind of self-judgment or negativity about your eating patterns, but start with awareness.

Food is pleasurable. So if you are feeling really down, having something that is both pleasurable and good for you is just a nice way to take care of yourself if done in a conscious way. Chewing a lot, breathing a lot, and communing with yourself, the food, and your family or friends helps create natural metabolic functioning in your digestion.

Chronic overeating accelerates the pace of aging and generally clogs up the works. It also doesn't feel as cathartic or comforting as we imagine it will. So it *is* something we want to be more and more aware of. And the practice on page 55, "Left Nostril Breathing for Healthy Eating," is a really gentle, sweet way to help rewire the habit without a whole lot of second-guessing and self-restriction. Also if you've suffered from eating disorders of any kind or just compulsive and chronic dieting, this practice is very medicinal to your system.

GLOWING SKIN TECHNIQUES

The best things you can do for your skin is drink a lot of water, eat alkalizing foods, get plenty of adequate rest and exercise, and use sunscreen on a regular basis—but here are a few other tips for good skin.

The health and integrity of your skin is a complete reflection of your internal health. If you have chronic blemishes, it's usually a sign of a weak liver. A mono diet of steamed beets and beet greens while drinking chamomile tea and water, no dairy, and no sugar will restore liver function while simultaneously giving you radiant skin with a really beautiful glow!

For women, if your skin is sagging and losing its radiance, this is a sign of poor vaginal muscle tone. I know, I know. You may have never heard that one before. That's because no one knows about it, except the yogis, Taoists, and tantrikas. But the firmness, the conditioning, and the tone of your facial skin are a mirror image of the tone of your vaginal walls. And there are simple yogic exercises to refirm, revitalize, and recondition the muscles in your pelvic floor, which ultimately affect your posture, your sense of self, and—you guessed it—your sex life. Similarly, a man's control over his ejaculation as well as the strength and circulation of the perineum and pelvic floor are deeply related to sexual function, prostate health, and urinary pressure with age. This is where the elementary yogic practices of body locks, or *bhandas,* have some very functional, householder uses.

Bhanda directly translates from Sanskrit to English as "lock" or "seal." And in a yogic practice, this lock refers to the isolation and contraction of certain muscle groups, essentially "locking" them. The uses of *bhandas* in a yoga practice (not including innumerable side-effect benefits) include:

- Locking an area of the body hydraulically to activate energy and pull energy up the spine

- As a method to smooth the path of the energy

- As a technique to seal energy in a certain area of the body—such as the heart, pranic reserve cavity (discussed later in "Fully Stress-Free"), or the system at large

- Activating shut-down chakras and circulating the energy effectively in the aura

- Adjusting and stimulating the glandular system for increased vitality and body wellness

Bhandas are foundational in Kundalini Yoga. And when we are getting specific and scientific about the way we want to apply *bhandas* to our lives, it is the use of the *mulbhand,* or root-lock, that has a direct enhancement effect on the firmness, luster, and youth of the skin. A simple tutorial on how to pull a *mulbhand* is included in the chart on page 61!

Another phenomenal yogic, homeopathic remedy is to use a yogurt douche.

Don't get me wrong about douching—any of those drugstore brand douches *are* really destructive to a woman's vaginal health. But natural douching is actually a very positive internal health practice. A toned and healthy uterus, vaginal walls, and pelvic floor will give you the same kind of health in the skin on your face and can also ultimately have an effect on fertility and hormonal balance through your chronological aging process. They will also save you from the hazards of urinary tract infections, kidney infections, and even yeast infections. The more you can keep yourself from taking antibiotics except when you really need them, the better for your whole system's health and longevity.

Yogurt is actually really fantastic for the skin in general. It cleans, tones, and firms it. You can massage yogurt into your face, then take a warm bath while letting the mask dry. You can also put a cup of yogurt directly into your bath. Another use is the following amazing yogurt-based body mask given by Yogi Bhajan for really glimmering results.

Above all, when your skin starts to dull, this is a sign to do more heavy *pranayam,* or breathing exercises. The 70 trillion cells in your body are naturally vibrant, dancing, and full of energy. This is the baseline state of every cell. What starts to happen with aging is, over time, our emotional toxicity, psychological toxicity, and material toxicity (from pollution, undigested denatured foods, drugs, and whatever else) start to dim this radiance with a kind

THE YOGURT DOUCHE

DIRECTIONS: In an at-home water douche kit (WaterWorks is a good brand), mix a tablespoon of yogurt with warm water and leave for a day. At the end of the day, take a shower and use the douche per package instructions. This is great to do before and after your period or, if you are postmenopausal, after sex, or just when the rhythm feels right.

of buildup. The cellular buildup blocks the inherent energy of the cell, which accelerates the aging experience.

The pranic molecules that come in on the breath act like little scrubbing bubbles on each cell. These subatomic packets of energy go into the cells and, with the inherent motion of their frequency, clear out emotional, psychological, and material buildup on a molecular level. So you actually start to restore the natural scintillation of each cell by just removing the crud that was blocking it. And this creates the radiance of youth not only in your appearance but also in your mental and emotional experience. Now every internal and external cell can have the same expression of energy that it did when you were younger, before all the buildup set in. And there's not one person I've ever met whose rudimentary personality as a very young person wasn't more vibrant and expressed than how we become when the buildup of toxicity mentally, emotionally, and physically happens in aging. Just do one of the breath practices from this book consistently, and you'll see what I mean.

I make my Kundalini practice more powerful and more sophisticated by pulling *bhandas*, or body locks.

Jalandhara Bhand

Neck Lock

I always pull a light neck lock when meditating. For neck lock, the chin is pulled into the throat, creating length in the back of the neck. This guides more energy into my brain and opens up the crown chakra.

Uddiyana Bhand

Diaphragm Lock

Pulling a diaphragm lock advances and accelerates the power of your practice. To pull this lock, exhale at the end of an exercise, pull root lock (see below), and then pull your diaphragm up into your rib cage as if you are trying to make your stomach entirely hollow. This helps give you tangible access to the physical location of the soul in the body.

Mulbhand

Root Lock

I increase the power of my practice by pulling a root lock at the end of exercises and meditations. The method I use for pulling a root lock is to finish the meditation, inhale, and then squeeze up on the perineum, sex organs, and navel point as though it were a full pelvic Kegel. This seals all the energy from the practice into my system.

HANUMAN BODY MASK

DIRECTIONS: Combine turmeric, yogurt, chickpea flour (besan), powdered ginger, and a lot of lemon juice to make a paste, and massage it into your body. Massage it in and let it dry on your body. Then, wash it off with warm water. Let your body air-dry, and then massage your skin with almond and sandalwood oils. This will heal your skin, leaving it glowing, smooth, and smelling sweet.

NOTE: Turmeric stains clothing and towels, so use dark towels and clean the bathtub immediately after bathing with this mask. You can do this recipe without the turmeric if you're concerned.

VIBRANT HAIR

Hair is a special thing. In society, the lushness and fullness of your hair says a lot about how your body is functioning. Yogically, hair means a lot in many ways.

Hair maintains the body's electromagnetic field and acts as an antenna for the aura (think *Avatar* movie). Hair is the only instrument that directly feeds vitamin D from the sun straight into the brain. The brain needs more vitamin D than any other organ of the body. This kind of concentrated solar energy also stimulates the pineal gland, the gland of enlightenment. So as part of yogic practice, hair has a very special place.

In Kundalini Yoga you see a lot of practitioners letting their hair grow to its fullest length. This is because uncut hair collects *energy* and acts as a shield and extension of your nervous system. However, you can practice Kundalini Yoga with any length of hair.

That said, we're interested in keeping our hair beautiful because it is an important part of our living system. And actually, the more care and conditioning you do for your hair, the more it helps in the yogic sense as well. Gorgeous hair isn't just good-looking. It also holds and resonates *energy,* and *that's* what makes it attractive.

For really luscious locks, try the three hair-care tips below.

If you are experiencing hair loss or hair breakage, that's a hormonal-glandular-metabolic system issue. It has nothing to do with how fast or slow the metabolism is. It means the body is not breaking down the proteins that you need or effectively delivering them to the right places. The body is a veritable genius, so if it's making a mistake like this, that means there is a block

TOP THREE YOGI HAIR-CARE TIPS

1. As per Yogi Bhajan, the Kundalini Yoga master, hair should be washed every 72 hours. Scalp secretions left unwashed on the head for any longer than that will irritate the nervous system, taking away from your natural beauty.

2. Never comb or brush your hair while it is wet. This stretches your hair shaft and causes breakage. Instead, let your hair dry naturally, soaking up solar energy. Then use a natural-bristle comb or brush to detangle your hair, distribute oils, and care for its electromagnetism.

3. Oil your scalp and hair shafts with almond and sandalwood oils prior to washing and then shampoo as usual. This will leave your hair shiny, strong, and smelling delicious.

somewhere. If your hair is breaking and thinning, take one of the yoga sets I give in the center part of the book, and practice it on a regular basis.

For any lack of vitality—including early graying of hair, sluggish metabolism, or dry or lackluster skin, I love the Kundalini Meditation to Regain Youthfulness given on page 65.

INNER BEAUTY VS. INHERENT BEAUTY

There's been a backlash against the idea that there are only certain kinds of beauty. The wellness and beauty industry is weaving a new narrative of inner beauty compared to its former focus on external beauty only. This, however, can also become another consumer-driven externalization of what beauty actually is. And on the other side of the polarity, there is spiritual rhetoric that claims you can just ignore the idea of physical beauty because you are inherently beautiful on the inside, which is also absolutely true. The beauty of a kind, compassionate, generous soul and mind is incredible and definitely more long lasting than running after Forever 21 consciousness.

But I'd like to evolve the conversation of what it means to be beautiful, past the polarity of inner and outer beauty. When the yogis say that everyone is beautiful, their words go beyond the external symmetries or pretty souls or deeds. They are referring to an *energy* of beauty, one that can be recognized and cultivated.

There is energy to beauty, a *frequency,* and it's inherent in your human birthright to behold it, live it, and embody it. This is the energy of your life force. As much as you are alive, you will, just by the nature of your human design, radiate a frequency of beauty.

How clear and how strong the frequency is depends upon your ability to let it radiate unimpeded. A good diet, a cleansed subconscious, and clarified cellular health will allow this intrinsic, fundamental energy to emanate

MEDITATION TO REGAIN YOUTHFULNESS

NOTES: This meditation achieves youthfulness of your skin, regenerates muscles, and makes gray hair disappear. The positive effects of this meditation are that it promotes a healthy sex life and a good diet. Our saliva is a powerful endocrine secretion that carries antibodies and proteins that increase health and youthfulness. That's why *chewing* your food is such a powerful practice.

POSTURE: Sit in easy pose, hands on your knees with the tips of your index fingers and thumbs touching. Roll the tongue backward in your mouth so that the bottom of your tongue is flat against the roof of your mouth. Begin sucking on your tongue. In a short time, a nectar-like taste will start to flow—just drink it.

EYES: Closed and focused at the brow point.

BREATH: Breathe normally.

TIME: 3 minutes, 11 minutes, or 31 minutes. Increase the length of time with practice.

TO END: Inhale, exhale, and relax.

unobstructed. And when this frequency is allowed to vibrate without impediment, you will look and feel beautiful. Unleashing, touching, and tapping your inherent innocence and goodness—the frequency.

Yogi Bhajan said, "A true master will be known by his or her vast and magnetic aura that looks like the sun and by their simple, direct, and down-

The beauty that you have within is most bewitching, but you are so afraid of relating to it. You have found a way out to relate to every other beauty but your own. Human is very bewitching to itself. Light is light and every human being has his or her own light, but instead of looking at your own light, reading your own book, living your own life, living your own house, guiding your own self, you look to others.

—YOGI BHAJAN

to-earth way." Like the phenomenon of light dancing on the surface of water, as long as there is water, there will be a glitter on the surface of it. As long as there is a physical form of you, there is a frequency of beauty that can and will radiate from you—if you allow it.

PROJECTIVE BEAUTY

So now you understand that your nature is inherently beautiful, and you have the techniques to deal with your cellular, glandular, and physical beauty. Your meditative mind accomplishments now can help you break out of the spell that says you can't stay luminous for as long as you are on this planet. However, I'm not promising that there's not going to be a day when you wake up and feel negative, insecure, or just a little bloated. I'm also not saying there will never come the day after you ate something weird the night before or you didn't exercise for a week and you feel a little heavy. Or you ate some sugar or fried food or whatever the thing is that triggers you about your physical experience in the body. I'm not promising that that morning won't come. It will, and it does. And that's okay. You can and will have those moments. For thousands of years, yogis and practitioners have taken advantage of technologies to radiate and project an appearance to the world. It's called *projective appearance*—something you'll want to command on the days when you don't feel your best.

When I was a kid, I was really into the Avalon book series by Marion Zimmer Bradley. I connected with Arthurian lore in a palpable, trans-space and trans-time kind of way. One of the parts in the series describes the capacity for the priestesses of Avalon to change and transform their outward look by the simple power and "magic" of commanding their mind.

This is actually a very real faculty. Ancient yogis and tantrikas have been described as being able to do the same thing. This may sound a little woo-woo, but I'm telling you, this self-knowledge is very *useful*!

If you have to show up somewhere and you're not feeling so hot but you want to be able to amplify your own radiance beyond neurosis or insecurity, you can absolutely do that! You can restructure your projective appearance to look like whatever you want, and people will see you that way.

We are living in a world where women are compulsively running around doing everything they can to not age. The fear is so deep, and the suffering is so deep. There have actually been a number of scientific studies about how people who are getting a lot of Botox are no longer having the same emotional spectrum due to the loss of nerve and muscle function in the face and vagus nerve. Because your brain and the chemistry of your endocrine system are connected to the way your face moves and your lips move, the mobility of your face directly impacts the full psychological and emotional range of a human being. So when you freeze your face, you don't experience your fullest human emotional spectrum.

Hollywood and the rest of the media world make billions of dollars off of the dysmorphic relationship we have with our bodies. But when we begin to realize it and start to practice a technology where we can practice and project how we physically, mentally, and energetically imprint our lives and the people we come into contact with, and therefore, appear on any day at any time in a way that feels empowering. That kind of positive projective power is real power.

Your projective appearance mostly comes down to clearing stress from the body-mind system and commanding your mind and energy in a positive imagination of yourself, even if that's not the way you feel at the current moment.

YOUR STRESS PERSONALITY

In Kundalini Yoga, we talk a lot about what Yogi Bhajan called the "stress personality." A stress personality is essentially what happens when, in time and through practice, you become so sympathetic dominant in your nervous system that you actually *become* a different person. It's you, but it's not you. It's the Dr. Jekyll version of you.

The stress personality has a whole *different face* than the tranquil, normalized, parasympathetic, dominant you. The urban dictionary slang for this is *fache* and I love how it describes the visual difference in you when you're in the Stress Personality. It means essentially that something is going on so hard core in your stress personality that you don't even *look* like yourself. At all. It's not your face—it's your stress fache. Or, even more descriptive, it's your "resting bitch face."

The musculature is different, and the vibrational projection is different. With all of that, even your genetics are different because stress turns off certain parts of the DNA and activates other strands. So it's not even the same genetic expression through the face. It's pretty wild. And so many of us live almost completely in our stress personality.

It's difficult to command your projective appearance when you are habitually stressed out. But if you have the wherewithal and tools to toggle into your relaxed, neutral mind quickly and efficiently, you can have the energy, intelligence, and skill to project differently from your physical and mental/emotional being. Even if you still don't have the energy in that moment to craft a projected appearance for the day, this relaxation creates in you what is known as the shield of grace.

Yogi Bhajan described the massive power of grace as, "The shield of radiation or radiant shield which protects the pranic balance in your entire living system, not only with you, and within you, and within your psyche, but how you correlate to all other psyches in your communication of memory . . ." Essentially, calm, humane, elegant composure protects the radiant and attractive energy of your entire living system. Not only does this shield protect you, but it also lets you communicate your inherent beauty and vitality to all around you.

When you have grace it doesn't even matter if you have the capacity to project or not. Anger and frustration start to clear out, your face starts to

BEDITATION

POSTURE: As soon as your alarm goes off, sit up in easy pose in bed or throw your legs over the side of the bed.

EYES: Keep your eyes closed, gently focusing up and in at the brow point.

BREATH AND MANTRA: Connect to your breath using long, deep breathing. Mentally chant *Sat* on the inhale and *Nam* on the exhale, vibrating the mantra at the brow point.

TIME: 1 to 3 minutes

TO END: Inhale, exhale, and relax.

shine, and the structure of your face shifts into one that is more innocent and therefore younger looking. So shifting out of neurosis into relaxation is true power, and the best way to facilitate this shift is to start with a practice first thing in the morning. You may have noticed that people who have some sort of daily mind-and-body training practice tend toward looking younger than their age.

For most of us, when we wake up in the morning, the mind has some kind of negative, dreading thought like, *F-ck, I don't want to get up today,* or some version of self-hating thought forms. And it's this first thought that, if you don't have some practice to change it, sets up your vibration for the whole day. And you might have a perfectly normal day. But underneath it all, your subconscious mind is running the preestablished negative thought form, which is creating stress and some version of the stress personality.

So to have a morning practice that resets your mind and your body back into a more healing and enjoyable wavelength is incredibly practical on many levels. Any of the practices given thus far in the book will help flip you into a more vitalized psyche. However, if you find that you really don't have the energy or wherewithal to get yourself to do a meditation when you get up each morning, you can do what I call beditation.

THE MAGIC OF AVALON

In reality, your physical body, the 70 trillion–plus cells that make up your body, looks and feels the way it does because your mind holds it that way. The cells of your body stick together and cluster based on the flow of your consciousness. This whole material *world* is actually a projection of our individual and collective mind stream. So your body, your physical body, can totally *reform* based on the projection of your mind.

In this world, nothing is static. Nothing is fixed. I would say it would take a lot of yogic power for you to grow six inches of height if that's what you wanted, but it's certainly not impossible. I've seen people grow a couple inches pretty easily, namely from unlocking their spinal health. Your whole physical form is a projection of your mind, which means your whole physical form can—and *does*—change based on your consciousness. And if you are *consciously* conscious of that, then you can have more direct control and influence over it.

Now, what the priestesses of Avalon and the ancient yogis and tantrikas were doing was a little bit different. They were projecting through their auras, a special aspect of the aura called the circumvent force.

Your sixth body, the arcline, affects a lot of different experiences in your life. (I go over it more in depth in other chapters—"Sweet Relations,"

SET FOR STRENGTHENING THE AURA

1. Place yourself in a downward-facing dog position (in Kundalini Yoga we call this triangle pose). Raise your right leg straight back and up. Begin a kind of push-up while keeping your leg up, exhaling and bending your arms to bring them near or to the ground. Inhale and return to the original position. Continue for 1½ minutes, switch legs, and repeat.

2. Come sitting in easy pose. Stretch your left arm forward, palm facing to the right. Cross your right arm under and over the left, attempting to grab your left hand from behind. Lock your fingers over one another and then inhale. Raise the arms in a straight line up to 60 degrees, as though they are extending out from the brow point. Arms do not come overhead. Exhale back to heart center. Keep your elbows straight. Breathe powerfully and continue for 2 to 3 minutes. Inhale, stretch up your arms, and relax.

3. Staying in easy pose, bring both arms forward with your palms facing each other. Then inhale, with your arms back like you're going to clap the back of the hands behind your back, and on the exhale, swing them up and forward at the level of the heart center. When you swing your arms forward, make sure it's with a force like you are going to clap but you don't. Continue for 2 to 3 minutes. Inhale, hold your breath. Exhale. Relax and sense the energy circulation through more than just your physical body.

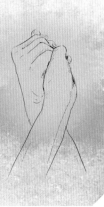

"Sex Is Science," and "Quantum Destiny.") The arcline has a way of interacting with your aura and all of your other energetic bodies to create a kind of weather pattern in your energetic field. This weather pattern is called a circumvent force.

When you command the circumvent force, you can create a powerful projection and the world will see you like that, no matter what you physically look like. Models and people in front of the camera professionally have this innate skill or practiced mastery of projecting certain energetics into the picture or broadcast to create physical, emotional, and psychic effects.

You can learn to do this too. One of my favorite yoga sets is the Set for Strengthening the Aura. It's a short and sweet set that's actually a great workout. It tones the musculoskeletal system, heals the internal organs, resets the glands, and improves self-esteem and self-assurance. Of course it also powerfully builds the aura! It's definitely one that will give you a true firsthand experience of working out your whole ten bodies simultaneously.

You know, you've seen women and men of all different ages who are just radiant beyond radiant or vital beyond vital. You know what it looks like. *Hopefully* you've had the chance to see it in yourself at some point. If not, I can assure you that these practices I have outlined will simply and effectively give you that experience. It's way beyond the size of your jeans that day. It's a vitalized, confident projection that you can practice, cultivate, and experience every day.

Ancient Tech 4. for SELF-HEALING

RA MA DA SA

You know how to heal yourself.

In ancient times, before modern medicine, there were higher mortality rates from the widespread contraction and rapid spread of different diseases. But there were also people who caught illnesses and lived. These are people who, by either education, intuition, or biological demand, understood they had the capacity to self-heal and quickly tapped into that flow. These people, for the most part, are the ones who passed on their genetics.

So you *know* how to heal yourself. It's coded deep into your ancient intelligence. It needs only to be acknowledged and turned on to start working. And the biggest problem with modern medicine today is that it doesn't acknowledge this very simple, very human, and very natural skill.

If you don't allow yourself to believe that you can heal yourself, your self-healing mechanism won't turn on or will only work in a limited way. If your mind is against you, if your mind cannot conceive of this ordinary and native capacity, you won't heal deeply—

or at all. This is a simplistic way of describing something that is much more complex, which I am not going to go into here, but it's useful to understand that you can train your mind and body impulses toward deep healing.

Kundalini Yoga connects you to your self-healing mechanism. It helps to turn it on and increases the wattage. There are so many techniques to jump-start this intrinsic capacity, and some are practically effortless. And this is exactly what is important to me in giving you these Kudalini self-healing practices: you know that you have options for your self-care and self-healing.

Whether Western medicine is important to you or you are more of a naturopathic sort—these practices can be incorporated into your regimen for maximum healing and long-lasting vitality. It's valuable, no matter what your stance is, to know the powerfully effective ways to take care of yourself and support your healing on all fronts, and on your own terms.

EATING AND IMMUNITY

Food is a powerful medicine. What you eat either contributes to your overall vibrancy, well-being, and longevity or impairs your natural rejuvenation, accelerates aging, and compromises your immune system. It's really very simple. Either the food you eat enhances and builds health, or it undermines it. Most people believe it's *what* you eat that creates health or disease. It's true that certain foods have immaculately healing compounds that create immense curative effects on the body. However, what you eat isn't half as important as how well you digest it.

For instance, dairy is a celebrated part of the yogic diet. Milk, yogurt, cheese, and ghee condition and strengthen the system. In India, for instance, cows are worshipped because of this dietary gift. That said, the baseline yogic rule on food is *don't eat anything that you can't digest in eighteen hours.* So if you know you can't digest dairy—it won't help you no matter how many Ayurveda books insist its health and radiance attributes are unparalleled.

Dairy is a hot dietary topic, and I am not getting into any nutritional dogma in this book. Anthropology can have a very big determinant on how you digest certain properties in certain foods. Also I am a huge fan of raw unpasteurized dairy if you're going to consume it at all. This makes the digestion process much easier and quicker and raw dairy maintains many traceable medicinal aspects.

So healthy food, its preparation, the dos and don'ts all are pretty hot news in the wellness scene, especially organic vegetables, gluten-free grains, and—if you're going to eat meat—grass-fed beef and other organic options. You can go raw, paleo, macrobiotic, whatever. Everyone is talking about what's "good" for you. But if what you eat doesn't exit your system in eighteen hours or less, *it's not working for your digestive metabolism.* This and other ethical and energetic reasons are why Kundalini yogis, including myself, choose vegetarianism and plant-based diets. However, like I said, I am not preaching any dietary dogma particularly.

I'm italicizing these teachings because *it's important to know and have choices.* If you can't digest your food in eighteen hours or less, then you are slowly fostering disease in your body. In these conditions, the system experiences a daily depression because it is overworking to digest the lingering food in your stomach. This accumulated toxicity potentially leads to an imbalance of some sort or eventually illness. And meat certainly is one of the big culprits of slow digestion, creating digestive buildup and related issues.

Most men and women in the West, even *children,* across ethnic and economic backgrounds have digestive issues. But this isn't just a modern problem. Ancient peoples also experienced digestive difficulty. This is because digestion is one of the first places to experience a breakdown when the body-mind-emotional-energetic system is under stress. As such, yoga—as the ancient science of human maintenance and growth—developed many techniques to heal and rejuvenate the digestive process.

A regular yoga practice will completely tone and reboot your digestive system. But if you need a little extra assistance, here is where the fun stuff comes in: recipes! Healing with food is such a powerful curative and medicinal tool for optimal health. And the results are so real and trackable. Also the process of picking, shopping, and creating with food is a healing process unto itself. For digestive cleansing, these two simple elixirs offer particularly amazing results.

If you are going for a full digestive recalibration, the following simple yoga pose will help balance your digestion.

TWO YOGI RECIPES FOR DIGESTIVE REBOOT

STOMACH AND INTESTINAL TRACT CLEANSER

Sauté 2 tablespoons to a ½ cup of finely chopped orange peel in olive oil. Mix in turmeric paste (turmeric powder that has been precooked in water). Take on an empty stomach in the morning; then throughout the rest of the day, fast on either water and juice or a mono diet. Repeat daily or as necessary.

GREEN CHILI ANTI-POISON INTESTINAL REMEDY

Blend green chilies with garlic and water. Take on an empty stomach in the morning and fast throughout the rest of the day on a mono diet. Repeat daily until digestion is healed.

ROCK POSE PRACTICE FOR DOUBLE DIGESTION

NOTE: Rock pose is very simple, and it's named this because it's said that while sitting in this position, you can actually digest rocks.

POSTURE: Sit on your heels, relax your hands on your upper thighs, and breathe.

EYES: Keep your eyes closed, gently focusing up and in at the brow point.

BREATH: Breath is long, deep, relaxed, and drawn into the lowest part of the lungs and the belly.

TIME: 1 to 11 minutes, or as long as you can

TO END: Inhale, exhale, and relax.

FOOD-BASED PHARMACY

Medicinal foods can be very simple and accessible wherever you live and whatever socioeconomic status you are currently experiencing. This is really one of my favorite areas of yogic skill sets because it's very alchemical. Intelligent use of food helps you stay healthy. In addition to being delicious, the right food can detoxify your internal organs, feed your glandular system, regenerate your creative and sexual energy, stimulate your immune system, and help clean and rebuild brain function as well as improve your entire nervous system. It's really a sophisticated approach to medicine, and it's potently effective.

Healing with food and herbs is an elaborate art. Ayurvedic and Chinese medicinal texts are thousands of pages long. But to simplify something very complex, food-based healing works like this: Plant and animal food products (such as dairy, honey, and meat) are composed of active molecular vitamin, mineral, and phytochemical configurations. These active molecules interact with the human body at a cellular DNA level to bolster, heal, and improve it—or on the flip side, to destroy it.

The science is complex. It's not just that vitamin C is good for you—although it's been shown in test tubes that no virus can withstand a vitamin C–rich environment. It's not that your nervous system needs sulfur to work or that celery provides an easily metabolized dose of that sulfur—although both are true. It's that the molecular—and dare I say, *energetic*—configuration of these foods supports the DNA in its integrity and in its improvement. And when the DNA is supported in unique and specific ways, and each food interacts with your DNA in a different way, the body can do all kinds of things, like fight internal fungi, bacteria, and viruses. It can rebuild artery walls in the heart and recondition all of your overtaxed organs. The body is an expert self-healing mechanism. It just needs the support.

Seeking command over food-based healing could lead you down the rabbit hole of eleven years of Ayurvedic study, but it doesn't have to. Being sensitive is really enough, because it is ultimately very intuitive. You know on some level what you need to heal. These foods and practices will help to open up your innate experience of that intuitive healing compass.

Because it's such a total cure-all, yogi tea is one of my favorite medicinal recipes. It's like a medicinal silver bullet. It is a true tonic to the whole system. Any illness or lingering virus you might be dealing with, yogi tea, in concert with a restorative mono diet, will clear it up. That's a promise. The benefits of yogi tea could fill pages. Here's how it's made.

heavenly yogi tea

For Each Cup:

10 ounces water (about 1⅓ cups)

3 whole green cardamom pods, cracked

4 whole black peppercorns

½ cinnamon stick

½ teaspoon black tea

½ cup milk (or almond milk)

2 slices fresh ginger root

Cooking Instruction:
Bring water to a boil and add spices. Cover and boil 15 to 20 minutes; then add black tea.

Let sit for a few minutes, add the milk, and return to a boil. Don't let it boil over. When it reaches a boil, remove immediately from heat, strain, and sweeten with honey if desired.

THE BREATH OF LIFE

One of the best ways to amplify your immunity and activate your self-healing mechanism is with your breath.

It's known that bacterial organisms, fungi, parasites, and viruses can't live in oxygen-rich environments. So if you are down and out with the flu, or if you have a more severe illness or cancer, you need to amp up your deep

IMMUNE SYSTEM BOOSTER: THE INNER SUN

NOTE: This advanced immune therapy attacks viruses and bacteria.

POSTURE: Sit in easy pose. Bend your left arm, raising your hand up to shoulder level. Face your palm forward and touch the tip of your ring finger to the tip of your thumb. Make a fist with your right hand, but keep your index finger out. Gently close off your right nostril with your index finger.

EYES: Keep your eyes closed, gently focusing up and in at the brow point.

BREATH: Breath is a steady Breath of Fire.

TIME: 3 to 11 minutes

TO END: Inhale deeply and hold the breath. As the breath is held, interlace your fingers just below your throat and try to pull your fingers apart. Hold the breath for as long as you can, then exhale. Repeat 3 more times. On the last exhale, shoot the breath out through upturned lips, with your tongue curled back on the roof of the mouth. Relax.

BREATH OF TEN MEDITATION
TO BECOME DISEASE-FREE

NOTES: This pranayam is a magnetic energy therapy. The energy connection between the hands must not be broken. It can give you a disease-free body and a clear meditative mind, and it can develop your intuition, but it requires practice.

POSTURE: Sit in easy pose with a straight spine. Relax your shoulders and bend your elbows to bring your hands to a clapping position at the level of the solar plexus. Move your hands in and out as if you are clapping, but don't actually let the hands touch.

BREATH: Inhale in 5 strokes through your nose as you "clap" 5 times. Then exhale in 5 strokes through the mouth as you "clap" 5 times again. Coordinate your breath with the motion of your hands. Continue and concentrate on the energy slowly building between your hands.

TIME: 3 to 11 minutes, gradually working up 16½ minutes if it interests you

TO END: Inhale, hold your breath for 20 seconds, and press your hands hard against your face. Exhale. Inhale again, hold your breath for 20 seconds, and press your hands hard against your heart center. Exhale. Inhale for the last time, hold your breath for 20 seconds, and press your hands hard against your navel point. Exhale and relax.

DOG'S BREATH

NOTES: This exercise brings energy to your immune system to fight infection. It is a very healing exercise. When you feel a tingling in your toes, thighs, and lower back, it is an indication that you are doing this exercise correctly.

POSTURE: Sit in easy pose or rock pose.

BREATH: Stick your tongue all the way out of your mouth and keep it out as you rapidly breathe in and out through the mouth in a panting diaphragmatic breath.

TIME: 3 to 5 minutes

TO END: Inhale, hold your breath for 15 seconds, and then press the tongue against the upper palate. Exhale. Repeat this sequence 2 more times.

yogic breathing. That's a simple way to increase the body's natural healing impulse.

Increasing your breathing doesn't just saturate your bloodstream with oxygen, thereby expunging diseased material from the body—it also increases the amount of prana in the system. Prana is life force. If you're sick, you're depleted in life force. Healing isn't just about food molecules and DNA and oxygen, it's about prana. And this is also why deep breathing and breath work are so effective in healing the physical and emotional bodies.

Western medicine is in a kind of tailspin right now. No one can find a cure for AIDS. Cancers are endemic. New viruses are coming all the time, mutating quickly. Antibiotics are no longer doing their job, and the overprescription of pharmaceuticals is heavily depleting our collective health. The normal way of researching a disease for thirty years and then crafting some complicated synthetic cure hasn't ever actually worked. It isn't holding up as the viral world rapidly spreads and transforms itself.

What the body requires is jolts of prana, continuous lifeline to free up infinite energy. And actually it's possible to get a lot of prana from fresh, organic plant foods. But the easiest, fastest, and most bio-available way to intake more prana is through your breath.

I personally practice some amazing breath pranayams for whenever I'm feeling as if my immune system is in jeopardy, or even if it's simply lagging a bit. I'm going to share a couple of my favorites here. You can do each practice for three to eleven minutes whenever you're feeling low on energy, when you feel a sickness is coming on, or when you are more seriously dealing with disease.

Having sensitivity to the breath is also a powerful way to know when you are going to get sick or develop an even more serious illness. Developing pranic awareness is actually one of the first habits of a yogi. Sensing disruptions in the pranic field, the field of life force that permeates the fabric of your personal space and time, will allow you to know something is off before it progresses into more serious illness or disease. The more sensitive and intuitive you become, the more specific you can get about how that disruption would manifest if allowed to continue.

Here is the best meditation for forging a relationship to the depth and power of your own breath and life force.

BREATH AWARENESS EXERCISE

POSTURE: Sit in easy pose with a straight spine, hands in gyan mudra.

EYES: Keep your eyes closed, gently focusing up and in at the brow point.

BREATH: Breathe normally.

MENTAL FOCUS: Let all of your attention gather on the breath. Sense the breath as a quality of motion. Bring your attention through the 1-inch square above your nose where the eyebrows meet. Then focus your attention through your brow down to the navel point area. Concentrate just below the interior of the umbilicus. Feel the motion and life energy of the breath. Visualize the body as luminous. As you inhale, the light increases in brightness, extent, and penetration. Let that breath and light merge with the entire Cosmos. Let the breath breathe you. Experience yourself as a unit and the Cosmos as unlimited. Feel that you are a part of that vastness. The breath is a wave on a much greater ocean of energy of which you are a part.

TIME: 3 to 11 minutes

TO END: Inhale, exhale, and relax.

SLEEP

Sleep is good. Very good. The body needs to sleep in order to consciously channel energy and keep your life going smoothly. And if you're not sleeping well, you know you're missing out on something.

Everyone has a different number of sleep hours they need in a night. And often we feel that number is higher than we actually need because of built-up fatigues and toxicities in the system.

Normally a very healthy body needs about five to six hours of sleep per night. In actuality anything over six hours is just time when the subconscious is dumping its overload, so this sleep is usually not deeply restorative because the subconscious mind creates dreamscapes full of fear and anxiety during this extra time. If you've ever woken up from a long sleep but were still exhausted, you know what I mean. It's better to wake after six hours and release the subconscious load in meditation. And then if you need another power nap during the day, you can follow some of the yogic power nap suggestions below.

It's actually *when* you sleep, as opposed to how *long* you sleep, that has the greatest impact on your vitality, health, and healing. Powerful, healing deep sleep occurs between ten at night and two in the morning. This is a time cycle when the organs rest, rebuild, and repair themselves. If you are not sleeping during these times, then all the intensity your body endures each day from work, pollution, and improper eating never gets a chance to get mended. This eventually leads to superficial illness, which isn't necessarily fatal but is nevertheless life sucking and chronic, or can even lead to something that actually is more malignant and carcinogenic. And if you are sick in any way at all and you are on a healing path, then putting yourself to bed by 10:00 P.M. is a definite must for regenerating your body.

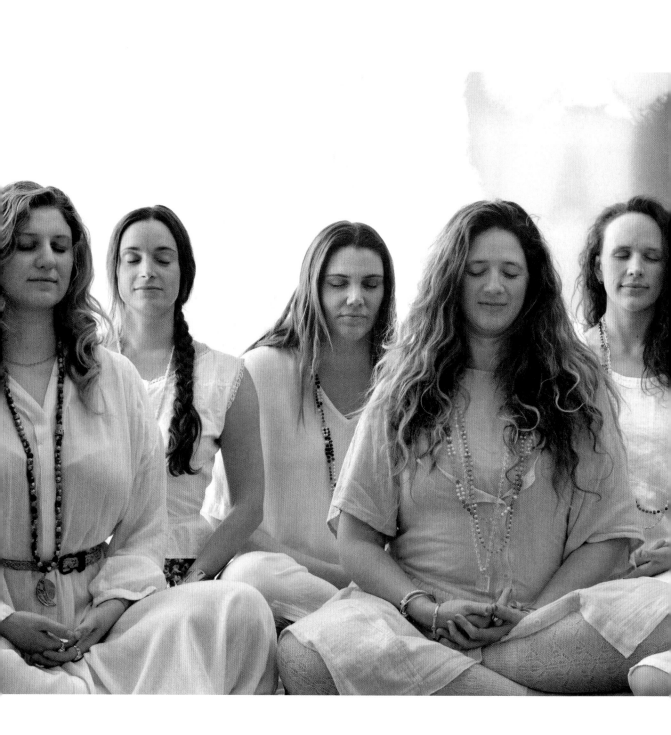

THE YOGIC POWER NAP

Yogi Bhajan said that a true yogi can put himself or herself to sleep almost on command. (Interestingly, he used this same verbiage to define what it means to be wealthy.) For those of us who haven't mastered the art of instant shut-eye, here are some yogic napping strategies.

- Before your nap, splash a bit of cold water on your face, hands, wrists, forearms, and feet. Cold-water hydrotherapy on these power points relaxes the nervous system and prepares the body for rest.
- Stretch lightly where you feel tight to trigger the body to release tension.
- Use a compass application on your smartphone to orient your body to sleep east to west. This sleep configuration recharges your energy field.
- Nap for a total chi cycle of 11 minutes.
- Nap to a recording of the gong. The sound of the gong purifies the subconscious mind and allows the body to relax more deeply. Recordings of Yogi Bhajan playing the gong are available online as well as gong tracks by the group White Sun.
- If you're still having trouble unwinding, block your right nostril with your index finger and breathe long and deeply through the left nostril. Left-nostril breathing triggers cooling in the body. Breathe this way until you feel happily dreamy.

HEALING INSOMNIA NATURALLY

If you are finding it difficult to go to bed at the hour you want to, or you wake up in the middle of the night and can't get back to bed, there are some tools to alleviate your insomnia. Insomnia is not a myth. Seventy-two million people suffer from insomnia every year, and almost half of the senior population in the United States faces sleepless nights.

So insomnia is a real issue. But what I'd like to discuss is the way we too often approach the condition and the treatment of it. When you see statistics that high it speaks deeply to a society that does not have the tools to deal with the everyday stressors and pressures they are facing. Not to mention that insomnia is a hugely profitable modern malady. Who profits? Well certainly not the people who are suffering from it. It's the pharmaceutical industry.

I remember reading this really alarming *New York Times* article some years ago with the headline "Record Sales of Sleeping Pills Are Causing Worries" that charted a 103 percent rise in prescriptions for insomnia medication.* *103 percent!* And that doesn't even count what was being purchased over the counter. This really got me thinking, if sleeping pills worked the way the drug companies say they work, then the prescriptions of sleeping pills should be going down, right? Because people are going to sleep and healing their insomnia—or did I miss the fine print? (*Yes, I definitely missed the fine print because all of these drugs have horrific side effects*.)

The pharmaceutical industry has a market share of around $1.6 billion from sleeping pills. They have a vested interest in you *not* being able to sleep. So let's just see the whole reality for what it is. Certainly stress is involved, so having a daily meditation practice will start to shift your sleep cycles. But more often than not, it's not just anxiety but also an actual physiological component that is blocking your sleep.

The pineal gland, a small gland the size of an apple seed that sits in the direct center of your brain, produces the hormone melatonin, which is in charge of regulating sleep cycles. When the pineal gland is healthy and clean, it is very photoreceptive. Though the pineal gland doesn't pick up light the

---

* Stephanie Saul, "Record Sales of Sleeping Pills Are Causing Worries," *New York Times,* February 7, 2006, http://www.nytimes.com/2006/02/07/business/07sleep .html?pagewanted=all&_r=0.

SHABAD KRIYA FOR DEEP SLEEP AND RADIANCE

NOTES: For maximum effectiveness, practice this meditation every night before bed. If you wake up in the middle of the night, just start the meditation again and continue until you fall asleep.

POSTURE: Do a little beditation and find a comfortable position in bed that allows the spine to be straight. Place your hands in your lap, palms up with your right hand resting in your left. Touch your thumbs together and point them forward.

EYES: Close the eyes nine-tenths and focus on the tip of the nose.

BREATH AND MANTRA: Inhale in 4 equal parts, mentally chanting the mantra *Sa-Ta-Na-Ma*. Hold the breath, vibrating the mantra 4 times for a total of 16 beats. Exhale in 2 equal strokes, projecting mentally *Wahe Guru*. This is the sound current of the pineal gland, and it means, in essence, "It's sublime to get enlightened." It's said that *Wahe Guru* is literally the sound that the pineal gland makes as it secretes, the way *pwop pwop* is the sound of a dripping faucet.

TIME: 15 to 62 minutes, or until you fall asleep

TO END: You will end naturally when you are sleeping.

same way as our eyeballs do, it does register illumination and darkness. And this very supple photoreceptivity gives it the sophisticated messaging it needs to release the luxurious melatonin secretions at the right time and in the right amounts.

So in a healthy brain, sleep is happening in a smooth, regulated way. However, most people don't have soft, receptive pineal glands. They have *calcified* pineal glands. And that happens from fluoride in drinking water, in toothpaste, toxic compounds in pesticides, and all other kinds of sources. It also is a by-product of unhealthy and rapid aging processes. You would do well to cut some of these items from your life. But we live in an increasingly toxifying world. You just can't control all the substances that come into your body all the time.

This is another reason why yogic technologies are so essential on the planet right now. We can't control what company is dumping what where or whether or not the food packager correctly labeled the organic chips if they were spiced with GMO pepper. It's really an insane task to monitor everything because you'll end up like the boy in the bubble. Even then you just can't control all the variables. But you *can* detoxify—powerfully and daily! And one of the best yogic meditations for decalcifying the pineal gland and restoring natural melatonin balances (so that you can sleep, and *heal*!) is the Shabad Kriya for Deep Sleep and Radiance.

This meditation creates relaxed, restorative sleep patterns; regenerates nerves; and releases the secretions of the pineal gland. And, because melatonin and the pineal gland also regulate tissue regrowth, the Shabad Kriya for Deep Sleep and Radiance also grows beautiful hair and skin. After a few days to months of practice, the rhythm of your sleep will be regulated, and this new, healthier rhythm will actually stay with you throughout the entire day, which is a very practical side effect. Stress will slowly leave your system, which allows your body and mind to heal more.

SACRED OUTLOOK

Illness, even just a twenty-four-hour cold, creates stress, because you need more energy to get through the day.

Stress impairs your ability to heal. Subconsciously we tighten when we have trauma. That tightening, on a physical level, restricts your circulation. Then your body has a much harder time healing itself. And this subconscious contraction happens on all levels of the ten bodies.

The ten-body system always wants to come back to a state of healing and equilibrium, but it can't do it quickly and fully with stress and tightness. If you can relax around the trauma or lingering stress in your body, the affected area of disease will begin to get oxygen and circulation, and will eventually heal faster.

I've worked a lot with burn survivors. The ones who didn't mentally and emotionally identify with the blistering of the skin healed faster and more completely. There was a study done proving this, and I can personally attest to its accuracy. Essentially, the people who had massive burn experiences but didn't go into "burn consciousness" minimized the whelping and damage to their skin.

So the less tension you hold around illness or traumatic events, the more you heal. The less bracing on a physical, mental, energetic, or emotional level, the more progress you can make. This kind of relaxation really requires what the Tibetan Buddhists call a sacred outlook.

A sacred outlook dictates that if you can see everything as sacred in your life—the most challenging to the most beautiful—your whole experience of life deepens and becomes more fulfilling. You have a choice to create elegance and self-healing out of the muck of your lineal patterns, genetics and neuroses. That act creates in actuality "the ground" that you walk on as a human being, as Chögyam Trungpa Rinpoche put it so eloquently. And we all have had personal experiences, or know someone who has, where a deep illness created the most profound sense of wonder and gratitude for life. That revelation occurs when you don't isolate the sacred to only what is convenient or positive or looks good.

Sacredness doesn't happen in some ivory tower of "good experiences." When only the "good" is sacred, it becomes separate. It becomes materialistic.

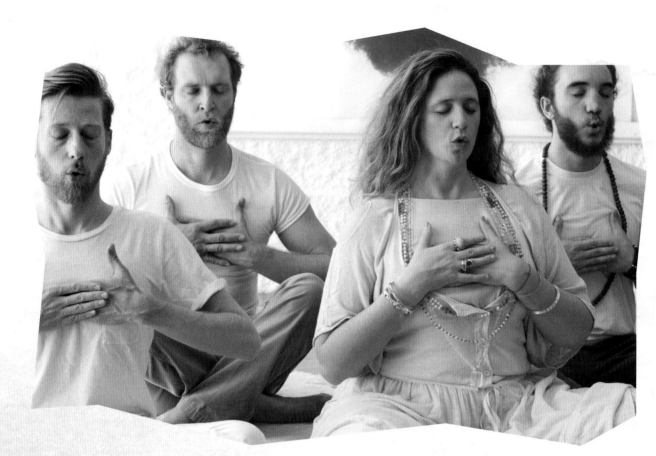

SELF-CARE BREATH

POSTURE: Sit in easy pose and place your hands on the center of your chest, left palm down and then right.

BREATH: Begin a steady, powerful Breath of Fire through a rounded mouth.

MENTAL FOCUS: Focus on the shape of your mouth, imagining the shape of the breath as a ring.

TIME: 5 minutes

TO END: Inhale and hold the breath, mentally repeating, "I am beautiful, I am innocent. I am innocent, I am beautiful." Exhale through the nose. Repeat 5 times. Relax.

Sacredness is in the every moment. And every moment isn't pretty. Some-times, even with the most precise intuition, you don't know what life is going to throw at you. Or you could see it coming and still not be able to stave it off. That *is* life and part of the cycles of experience. It's not always going to be easy or fun. But with a sacred outlook, you are training yourself to be a true practitioner of human wisdom and dignity in every moment of your life.

Sometimes, when doing really deep spiritual and physical detoxification, you end up going through a healing crisis of some sort. This is indicative of something actually getting cleared through your practices. It's good news, even if it doesn't feel like it.

Good. Bad. Up. Down. Crazy. Serene. Glorious. A total shit show. It's all sacred. It's *all* sacred. And cultivating this level of acceptance, appreciation, gratitude, acknowledgment, neutrality, and grace creates the relaxation and strength you need to allow fundamental and life-changing healing.

One of my favorite meditations for establishing a baseline of sacred ap-preciation is this Self-Care Breath. The bonus is that it heals and strengthens your nervous system. Stress happens even without our conscious participation. When you strengthen and balance the nervous system, you stay tranquil and relaxed despite the level or speed of stress input.

CONNECTING TO THE COSMIC HEALING FORCE

Yogi Bhajan said this about self-healing:

> *The process of self-healing is the privilege of every being. Self-healing is not a miracle, nor is self-healing a dramatization of the personality as though you could do something superior. Self-healing is a genuine process of the relationship between the physical and the infinite power of the soul.*

I feel like this really distills it. Self-healing isn't some kind of piece of science fiction. It's normal. It's your birthright. At the same time, it can be completely cosmic.

Healing involves the power of the infinite. And the infinite is one of those mind-boggling realities that can only be experienced and wielded. It cannot be explained or conceptualized, as that immediately creates a distance between you and your most infinite power. In what is really going to be the biggest victory of this new era, the power of the infinite is more and more recognized as not outside you, but deep within you. We are not completely there yet, but more and more people are turning within to experience the phenomenon of God, previously known only as an external figure that had to be connected with via a human in some power position or other religious construct.

The millennial generation is trailblazing an exodus from organized religion. And this is the beginning of a more massive shift in how we relate to infinity, the Universe, ourselves, societal power structures, and each other.

There is an immensely powerful mantra for self-healing and the healing of others called Ra Ma Da Sa, and it harnesses this infinite and intimate link. These sound codes are just like area codes. When your mouth, tongue, and vocal cords resonate them, you are almost literally dialing up a vibrational line to resonate the whole system with a higher healing field.

With Dr. Emoto's groundbreaking work of showing how sound and certain phrases changed the molecular structure of water, so too these mantra sound codes change the molecular structure of your system made up of more than 70 percent water. I'll be going deeper into the science of sound later, but for now try this syllabic mantra to help you and anyone you focus on receive instantaneous healing, peace, and calm.

RA MA DA SA HEALING MANTRA

POSTURE: Sit in easy pose if doing a formal meditation. The mantra can also be chanted at any time, anywhere, without creating a specific meditative setting. If chanting this mantra as a meditation, tuck the elbows into the ribs and bring the forearms up, close to the body. Now, bend the hands back, away from the body and stretching the wrists, angling the hands 45 degrees out to the side. Keep the palms very flat, as they will start to accumulate healing energy.

EYES: Keep your eyes closed, gently focusing up and in at the brow point.

BREATH AND MANTRA: *Ra Ma Da Sa, Sa Say So Hung.* Breathe deeply and chant in monotone or in melody with a recording (a classic is the version by Snatam Kaur, and I'm partial to the recordings by Erin Breech on RA MA Records and by Gurujas of White Sun). Pull on the navel point as you chant *Hung.*

MENTAL FOCUS: Visualize the person or people who need the healing. Send the energy to them.

TIME: 3 to 31 minutes

TO END: Inhale deeply and hold the breath. Visualize the person you wish to heal as being totally healthy, radiant, and strong. See the person engulfed in white light and completely healed. Exhale and repeat 2 more times. Then inhale, stretch your arms up, and shake out your hands and fingers.

5. Fully STRESS-FREE

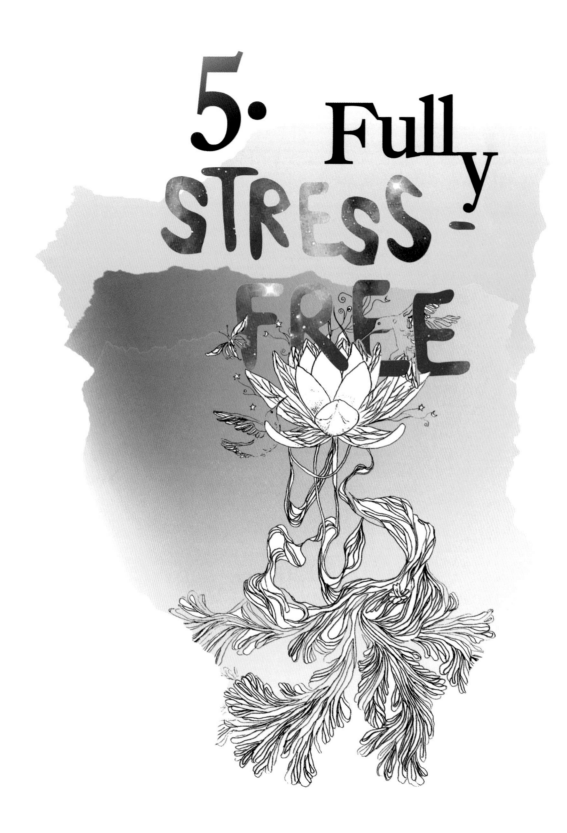

There's so much stress in the world. So much anxiety. So many depleted adrenal glands and so many fried nervous systems. Our modern life is demanding so much of us, and in many ways our physical and mental conditions are more and more taxed.

This level and consistency of deep stress contributes to a lot of dissatisfaction in life as a whole. It's challenging to find the joys in life, big or small, when there is a constant stream of deep panic about the future and the past running through you. And how can you be satisfied in life without some experience of happiness and joy on a daily basis?

There's a real need to develop the capacity to live in the pressurized world in a way that allows our systems to do what they actually do best when given the chance, which is to be happy, be healthy, be creative, serve others, and thrive. This is why yogic practice, in my opinion, is no longer a luxury. Yogic practice and lifestyle allow us to detox stress and develop a stamina for high-intensity situations. And the intelligent use of this yoga—and *intelligent* doesn't mean "hard" (it's actually quite easy and simple)—allows you to navigate life in the world in such a way that the stress triggers create little to no hardship on your mental, emotional, and physical systems.

Recently, a study came out that proved that the brains of meditators and yogis literally physically respond differently to stressors on the system. Furthermore, the stressors don't wear the brain's chemical response down to the point that there is brain fatigue and trauma. Note that this does not mean that the stressors are not going to occur—it means that the system can be trained to respond completely differently, which creates a different biochemistry in the body.

The best way to start to be in command of how stress affects you—to be sophisticated and savvy about living life—is to be sensitive to rhythms.

DEEP RHYTHMS OF PEACE

Everything has a rhythm.

Your body has a rhythm. Your job has a rhythm. Your partner has a rhythm, and your relationship has a rhythm. Even the place you live has a rhythm. When you can command the rhythm of life, you then have a more rhythmic experience, which is to say, a better experience. All of our unhappiness stems from being out of rhythm with nature, out of rhythm with the flow of our own energy. Stress and anxiety happen when the rhythm of *you* is *arrhythmic* with the environment you are in.

You can be *ahead of the rhythm,* i.e. ahead of yourself in time. So often you can see this in actual body language. When you see someone overextending their head and neck out away from the body, that's a physicalized symptom of being ahead of yourself in time.

You can also be *behind the times.* This has less of a postural manifestation and more of an intuitive, emotional one. You can *feel* when you are behind the times. You feel as though you keep missing the beat. It's an uncomfortable place to be because you can sense that you are not up to speed but you don't know what to do about it. And life and the opportunities and miracles feel always just out of reach or you can't hold on to them even if they get into reach.

Whatever the case, ahead of the time or behind it, you are not *in sync*. And when you are not in rhythm, then you start to feel the pressure of the misalignment. And that misalignment, that arrhythmia, is called *stress*.

This is why all ancient cultures built the day based on some rhythmic movement and breath in the morning. This goes across all time and all cultures. Because in order to build something strong and sustainable, the people, as a group, had to be in rhythm with each other and with themselves, with the earth, and with their surroundings.

We don't live in the kind of societies we used to, but we still need to care for the rhythmic nature of our beings. This is true if we want to live long, vibrant lives. (It's well-known that in India, tabla players—hand drummers—have the longest lives because their brains are connected to primal rhythm.) And it's even more true if we have any dream of building a new society where individuals have cultivated free thought and all that it entails in terms of heightened quality of life, where community is healthy and strong, and where we live in sustainable, interdependent harmony with our planet.

There are a lot of yogic techniques for getting into the tempo of both your internal rhythm and the rhythm of the world around you. Of all of them, one of the simplest is to just get out into nature.

GETTING INTO NATURE

If you align yourself every day with the electromagnetic field of the earth, you will experience much less neurosis. This is very clear when you go to places that have more of a daily connection to the earth. In communities where people live very close to nature, the baseline neurosis is much lower than it is in urban areas, suburban sprawls, or anyplace else that doesn't have a strong connection with the natural surroundings.

Taking a walk outside, getting in the sun, or taking in fresh air allows each of the 30 trillion cells in your physical body to align with the rhythmic frequency of nature. It's an energetic and subtle activity, but the psychomagnetic alignment happens instantly and without effort. Each cell in your body has its own intelligence, and collectively in their conscious intelligence, they sync up to the highest, healthiest, most radiant rhythm available as soon as it's presented to them. So getting into nature allows the cells to tune themselves to something more creative and more present right away.

Another way to re-rhythm your being in a powerful way is to get the bare soles of your feet on the actual earth at least once a day. Feet are one of the biggest conductors of electromagnetic energy and one of only three convergence points on the body for your seventy-two thousand nerve fibers. This is why we ask yogis to remove their socks while practicing yoga or meditation—it allows your body to conduct a higher level of energy and electricity.

When you place your bare feet on the ground, each of those seventy-two thousand nerve fibers uptakes the electromagnetic pulse of the earth, which makes you instantly calmer. You can alternatively bring your forehead to the ground once a day, which will align your pituitary gland, your intuition, and your glandular and hormonal balance with the pulse of the earth. This, however, doesn't have to be on the bare ground—you can even do this just on your yoga mat or beside your bed in the morning in child's pose.

Grounding by connecting your bare feet with the earth is also a powerful way to develop nervous system strength and a parasympathetic nervous system dominance! When your parasympathetic nervous system is dominant, you can instantly self-soothe and switch gears from go mode to relaxation in a matter of breaths. This may seem simplified, but actually it is a very powerful tool that Kundalini Yoga technologies begin to develop in you as a baseline.

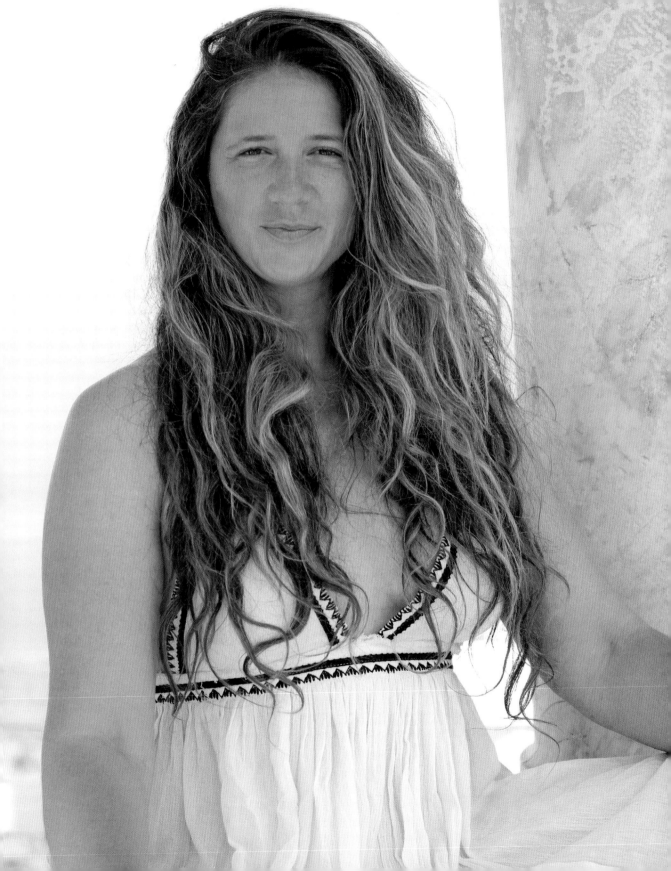

A QUICK-AND-EASY PRIMER ON THE NERVOUS SYSTEMS

Your body has three nervous systems that work together for your whole physiological, emotional, sensory, and motorized experience of life to happen. There is the central nervous system, which is composed of the brain and the spinal column. The central nervous system is your command center. And then there are two branches of your autonomic nervous system—the sympathetic and the parasympathetic. Your sympathetic nervous system triggers fight or flight responses. Your parasympathetic nervous system commands the rest, relaxation, and rejuvenating experiences.

Because of the highly pressurized state of the planet today, most of us live in sympathetic nervous system dominance. And the sympathetic nervous system dominance creates some of the major imbalances in us. It means that we are very much in this fight-or-flight, or "see bear—run from bear" space, and *a lot of times* that's happening even when *there is no bear.*

This constant fight-or-flight state wastes energy and puts a tremendous amount of stress on the system, which ultimately creates, over years, disease in the body and disease in the mind. And the modern diseases that we're dealing with, both in the body and the mind, are not diseases that our ancestors dealt with thousands of years ago. These diseases are accumulations of mental and emotional toxins triggered by the constant fight-or-flight experience in our nervous systems, and therefore hormonal and glandular systems respond with the same toxemia of stress response.

It's part of our capacity as humans to be able to move through the nervous systems at will. We want to train our systems to be parasympathetic dominant, which means we confront issues and obstacles effectively because we're calm and efficient and we don't let our stress get the better of us. If you're really healthy and have command of your nervous systems, you will be able to put yourself into a nap between nine seconds and a minute. Nine seconds to put yourself into parasympathetic dominance! Which means that you are able to maneuver through your nervous systems in such a way that you can contain and cultivate your energy throughout your day and your life.

ESSENTIAL STRESS-FREE TECHNOLOGY

Armpits

The armpits are the conjunction of your body's three nervous systems, hence the yogi saying, "If you get in the *shit,* you have to get in the *armpit.*" A really good trick for re-triggering yourself into parasympathetic dominance is to massage, stretch, and put cold water on your armpits.

Most people don't know how much the armpit has to do with nervous system balance. And because of the bras women wear and the constrictions on what's considered a normal use of the body—we sit in chairs, we don't move from our desks, we sometimes get up and walk, and *maybe* go dancing on Friday night but don't actually move the body through its full range of motion—the armpits don't get the attention they deserve. So it's really easy to build up stress and blockage there. Added to that are the toxic, chemical-laden deodorant options commercially available that clog up the lymph nodes in our armpits and cause even more modern disease and issues with brain function.

It's good to start the day with a cold shower or, if you just can't get your mind around that, even simply splashing cold water on each armpit for a good fifteen seconds or more. Then you start to train nervous system strength. If you get into a really stressful situation at work or somewhere in your daily life, you can duck into a bathroom and literally just massage the inside of your armpits with your thumbs for one to three minutes. I know this sounds somewhat ridiculous, but just try it. You will be shocked at how quickly you get a burst of energy and feel better. You can also grasp your elbows and stretch your arms overhead, really pulling on the armpits. Stay in this position and breathe for one to three minutes.

Food

Modern living can do a real number on your nervous system, especially if you are not watching what you eat. One of the wars for your mind is a nutritional war, which is why Monsanto and the whole GMO situation has been such a concern. It's been known for a long time that if your body is not functioning properly, you are easier to manipulate. And you actually have more of a tendency toward panic, anxiety, anger, and violence if your body is in a highly acidic state. This is why when you go into a low-economic neighborhood, you cannot find health food anywhere. That's not a coincidence; it's absolutely intended to keep a group of people from the clear mind and healthy body that they could achieve with fresh, healthy food.

If you create a blood balance and an endocrine balance and an organ balance and a hormone balance, then your body can actually handle a higher frequency of energy output for longer periods of time. Look at any professional or even hobby athlete—there's major dietary training that goes along with the strengthening and pacing of your mental and physical condition for utmost performance. You can handle more stress, and you can handle more goodness. So if you're someone who has chronic anxiety or suffers through semiregular panic attacks, you absolutely need to adjust your diet.

Sugar, caffeine, processed and packaged foods with gluten or weird ingredients, anything with hydrogenated oils—they all have to go because these foods create massive nerve degeneration and deterioration. Sugar is literally one molecule away from the same chemical configuration as methamphetamines. So the glucose spikes create instability in your mood, brain, and blood chemistry, and then they make you addicted to the highs and lows.

There's a whole science to eating for your nervous system. But to keep it simple, you are going to want to incorporate more cooked vegetables and *lots* of healthy fats. This is going to keep you grounded and your brain functioning optimally. In fact, any kind of root vegetable or spice (like carrots, beets, potatoes, sweet potatoes, lotus, yucca, yams, ginger, turmeric, onion, shallot, or garlic) will heal and ground your nervous system while providing you with sustained energy.

Yogis divide food into three categories:

SUN FOODS: Those that grow more than three feet above the ground, like avocados, cherries, nuts, and so on

GROUND FOODS: Those that grow within three feet of the ground, like beans, rice, green vegetables, and so on

EARTH FOODS: Those that grow underground, like potatoes, turnips, beets, garlic, onions, and so on

For nervous system healing, you'll want to create a diet of mostly ground and earth foods.

Celery and cucumber juices are immensely powerful when it comes to rebuilding the nervous system. If you've had panic attacks for years, or if you've done drugs or taken some kind of prescription medication that degrades the nervous system, celery and cucumber juices do major nerve regeneration. It's a good idea to incorporate a glass of organic celery or cucumber juice daily on an empty stomach. Then eat a mono diet of some sort of naturally green foods for the day. You will experience a difference right away.

Detoxing Stress

If you live in the modern world, chances are, you're deeply adrenal fatigued. The pressure is *on* in an intensely demanding way. Day-to-day life demands

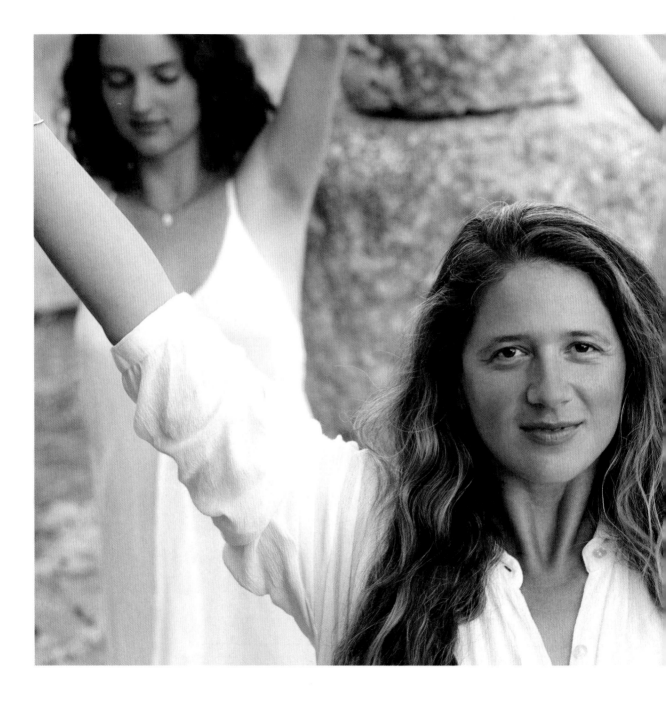

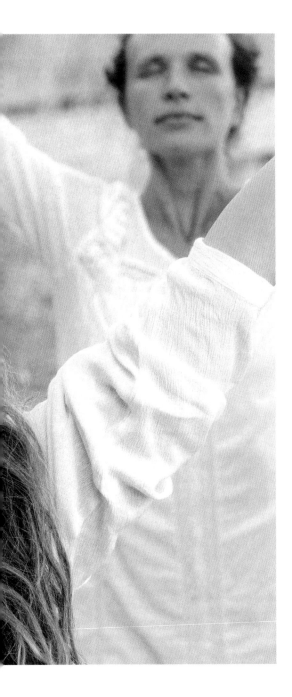

It's important to detox the stored hormonal remnants of stress so that we can get back to a place of balance and normalcy.

so much of us. When you're already exhausted, even just *driving* can be the stressor that sets off a toxic chain reaction in the body. Just *daily* living at this time on the planet is requiring more of us as humans than ever before.

Our adrenals are so taxed, and then we add caffeine and sugar, and drugs or whatever substances we think are helping us or taking the edge off, but actually they are only depleting us. Add in the habitual ways we engage in relationships with our emotional and commotional tendencies. Add our addiction to technology. Add all the ways that we drain ourselves. And then we are getting even more and more *depleted*.

We get irritated. And then we get impatient, and then we get angry. And then we just start to feel bothered by everyone, and then we start to treat ourselves and others in a less than compassionate way. You can see how we've created some terrible situations for ourselves, our species, and the planet, with irritable people acting irritably toward other irritable people.

We have such a waste dump of stored cortisol and other stress hormones in the body that consistently circulate the stress experience. That's why the body registers stress even if we're not experiencing new stimuli. When the blood is not clean, it's not possible for you to hold higher frequencies of energy.

We have a physical body so that you can move through the physical landscape with joy, fun, pleasure, and empowerment. If we want to experience these sensations, our body needs to be strong, healthy, and vitalized. And to get our body strong, healthy, and vitalized, our blood needs to be clean.

So it's important to detox the stored hormonal remnants of stress so that we can get back to a place of balance and normalcy. We're so stressed in our society that we don't even know what baseline human normalcy looks like or feels like for the most part. But we have the power to self-clean our blood and steer the body toward releasing old stress residue to restore natural blood chemistry. The most crucial place to start is with the kidneys and adrenals.

The kidneys filter waste from the blood and balance the fluids in the body. If there's too much vitamin C in the blood, the kidneys have to discharge the excess vitamin C. If there's too much water in the body, the kidneys have to take care of it. If there's too much of any one hormone in the blood—whether it's adrenaline, cortisol, or testosterone—the kidneys are taking care of that too! When your kidneys are overtaxed, they have a harder time filtering out all of the unnecessary compounds in the blood.

The kidneys filter about 120 to 150 quarts of blood a day. That's about thirty gallons! That's a lot. And if you think about how much denatured food we eat, how we don't hydrate, how much pollution is in the air, and how many daily stressors we're dealing with on an hourly and momentary basis, you can see how easy it is for the kidneys to get backed up. So it's important to care for these organs that do so much work without you even knowing or thinking about it.

At the same time, your adrenals—the tortilla chip–shaped glands that release the stress hormones adrenaline, aldosterone, and hydrocortisone (a.k.a. cortisol) into your bloodstream—sit on top of the kidneys. Whenever you work the kidneys, the adrenals detox and reset as well. This adjusts the adrenals to secrete these stress hormones at a less frequent pace and in lower quantities.

Hydration is a big component of healthy kidneys and adrenals. The kidneys need a daily flush in order to keep from storing too much backlog. Cutting down on acidic foods, cigarettes, and other toxins also helps your adrenals and kidneys heal. Of course if you really want a major overhaul on your system, a Kundalini Yoga set or breath is so powerful. And one of the great benefits of kidney and adrenal work is that it is thoroughly de-aging. It literally takes the years off of your face, body, and mind in no time.

THE HYPOTHALAMIC-ADRENAL AXIS

Mantras aren't required for yogic practice, but it's important to know how they actually work. While I talk about mantras in a few sections of this book, here I want to cover some of the physical science of sound and mantras as well as how they affect the secretions of the adrenals and the whole endocrine

HEALTHY, HAPPY, HOLY BREATH

POSTURE: Sit in easy pose with your index finger and thumb tip touching. This mantra can also be chanted at any time, anywhere, without creating a specific "meditative" setting.

BREATH AND MANTRA: *Healthy am I, Happy am I, Holy am I.* Inhale through the nose and suspend the breath. Silently repeat the mantra 3 times. As you exhale, repeat the mantra out loud 3 times. Continue the breath pattern.

TIME: 3 to 11 minutes

TO END: Inhale deeply, relax the breath, and sit silently for a minute or two. Then inhale deeply, stretch the arms up over your head with the fingers interlocked, and pull the spine up. Exhale and relax.

system. You might not expect this, but using the lips, tongue, and vocal cords to chant a mantra directly changes the frequency with which your adrenals release stress hormones.

Your adrenals take their cue from the hypothalamus via the pituitary gland. When you experience a stress stimulus, your nervous system sends the message to the central brain, where the hypothalamus is located. The hypothalamus then sends the message to the pituitary gland (the master gland), and the pituitary gives the go-ahead to the adrenals. This all happens in a split second. But the chain of command starts with the hypothalamus. Which means that if you adjust, balance, and strengthen your hypothalamus, you can short-circuit the stress response.

The hypothalamus is located just on top of the brain stem and right above the *roof of the mouth*. This is why the physical mechanism of chanting and vibrating a mantra actually gives a major adjustment to the hypothalamus.

Yogic science knows that there are eighty-four meridian channels on the roof of the mouth. A highly coded mantra will tap those eighty-four meridians using the tip of the tongue in a kind of Morse code. The code is so specific, precise, and advanced, it's like a computer code that takes you to the most miraculous part of the Internet. Only instead it adjusts your hypothalamus to secrete more oxytocin and dopamine in the brain. It enhances the brain chemistry and rewires neural patterns—and instantaneously gives you the joy, calm, and clarity that those chemicals have been proven to produce in the human system.

This is why—and I say it a lot in this book—as devotional and spiritual as mantras can be and have been used in some traditions, the science of sound is real and transformative, and we are just on the crest of major advancement in this arena. Mantra sound codes act on your hypothalamus and your entire brain in a direct and powerful way. So a really good way to brake-check the stress response is by using a daily mantra. I give a few in this book, some more syllabic, some in a sacred science language called Gurmukhi, and some in English. The "Happy, Healthy, Holy Breath" I give on page 112 is more than an English affirmation practice and does wonders to relax and rejuvenate you rapidly. I love the buzz I get from practicing this breath! It makes you feel so good.

RESERVE FORCE

So you're healing your nervous system, changing your diet, getting out into nature, detoxing the bloodstream of remnant stress, and using a mantra, but eventually you're going to have one of those days—or weeks—when you'll need something extra. This is when you'll need what we call a reserve force.

If you're practicing some of the Kundalini Yoga technologies in this book, you will begin to notice your stress responses lessen in intensity and length of time. But life throws a lot of curveballs our way. And if you've been practicing and healing, you'll be in good shape for the day-to-day stuff. But you will need to build up a reserve force of energy to handle the bigger challenges that life has to offer us.

The pranic, or breath force, reserve is like a 401(k) plan of your life energy. Every meditation, every pranayam, adds to this pranic reserve force. Biophysiologically, this energy has an actual locality. It is stored just under your solar plexus. Just the awareness of this storehouse is really helpful because you can begin to sense when it's growing, which will give you instant self-confirmation and, perhaps more important, you also can tell when the reserve is depleting so you can add to it with more conscious breath and meditation.

When we are out in the world, the pranic reserve gives us what is called in Tibetan Buddhism *Prajna,* which means space or clarity. It gives us space from reactions, space from our commotions, even space from certain karmic accumulations. So instead of *reacting* right away and setting off a chain of events, your reserve of energy kicks in and gives you *the commodity of clarity,* which allows you to change your action and change the course of activity quickly and directly to something that will be more positive and more beneficial to you and to others.

WORKING MOMENT TO MOMENT

All of these techniques will add to this reserve and give you access, so you can put "money" in and get "money" out. It's an ATM of your own reserve supply of energy. It gives you amazing power to be aware of ways you can gather and activate more energy in your system, which is so important as we are participating in a time when these stores need to be consciously used and replenished in a daily, hourly way due to the increase in demand and pressure in our everyday lives.

So all these techniques help us gather more energy and be able to utilize it in the most efficient way possible. Deeply and with little effort. Kind of like how much effort it takes to refill the gas tank in your car. You have to do it, but it's not something you usually fret about or feel like it's hard or impossible. It's just part of the cycle of your day and week.

Ultimately, everything has a rhythm. Your negativity has a rhythm. Your neurosis has a rhythm. And your *enjoyment and fulfillment* have a rhythm. How do we relate to our momentary life with more energy, more wherewithal, more compassion, more human beingness, and more fun? Take it one step at a time, or one breath at a time, and you will naturally begin to find a rhythm that creates more peace in you and your life. Once you're in this rhythm, it affords more presence and the true, deep experiencing of a lifetime. It sounds extremely simplified, but everyone dies, and *very* few people actually have the discipline and energy to actually *live*—to enjoy and cherish this life, no matter the ups and downs.

6.
BALANCED
Emotions

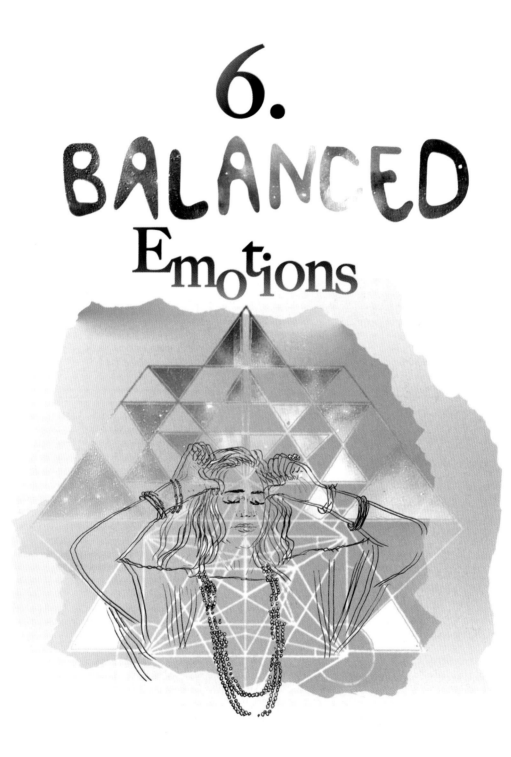

Emotions are just energy. But often it feels as if our emotions are running us. We're happy, we're sad, we're annoyed, we're in a rage. This is commonly considered normal human experience. We are humans, so there *is* a lot of energy in our emotional beings. But this emotional pendulum swing is not required to be fully in your human experience. Such an experience actually keeps you from your greatest level of fulfillment. Yogically, this kind of mood swinging is called *commotionality*.

And we live in a society that hypes moodiness and commotionality as normal human interactions. Between reality TV, soap operas, and social media, we are inundated with messages about the messy, crazy, emotionally spastic norms of human experience. And at the same time, there is a stereotype of spirituality where spiritual people are so even-keeled that they are somewhat boring and robotic or even a bit wet noodle-y. There is, however, a middle path of utter connectivity to your emotional energy spectrum, a deep sensitivity and awareness that allows you to hold on to energetic space as a buffer from habitual reactivity. Sounds too good to be true, right?

Well, emotions *are* your feelings. *Commotions,* however, are the disharmonious relationships with your feelings. Emotions are just like a rain cloud passing by. Rain clouds are a natural function of atmosphere and weather. Every once in a while, one will occur. That's just normal weather cycles. And beyond the clouds, the sun is always shining. Not to be cliché, but it's one of the environmental constants of this planet, even during the night. This is the same for your constant connection to steadiness and energy in life. And that connection, particularly with the remembrance of that connection in challenging or triggering moments, gives you the buffer of awareness and choice.

Our commotions are the freak-outs we have about the rain. It's the whole song and dance about the rain cloud and how it's going to ruin some aspect of your current day or life. It hasn't even started raining yet, but we're still making a huge to-do about it. That's commotionality, and it's how most people relate to their emotional spectrum.

Again, emotions are just pure *energy.* So if you can, in a moment, relax yourself, see a rain cloud, and determine, *Okay, a rain cloud is passing by. You know, it's nature. It could rain—it could be all sorts of things. Let's inhale . . . exhale . . . and, oh wow, look at that—it's actually beautiful. And now it's passed . . . and eventually it's sunny again.* That's right—you could experience the rain cloud directly and instantaneously as beautiful and useful. If you related to your emotions that way, think about how much more energy there would be in a day to do the things you know you have to do before you die.

What if you used the energy of your emotional being to propel forward as a leader, as a creative, and as a person inspired to live whatever you came here to live?

When you recognize that your emotion is just energy, you can utilize that energy in a way that might be beneficial to you *and moreover* beneficial to all of humanity.

BIOELECTRICITY OF EMOTIONS

One of the challenges to being skillful about how you are going to use your emotional energy is an ingrained magnetic patterning in your psyche and mind. Your psychomagnetic field is like a weather pattern that *you* have to live in and, unfortunately or fortunately, the people closest to you and anyone who spends time with you throughout a day also have to live in it. Your psychomagnetic field goes through all the normal weather fluctuations, but when your psyche is in harmony, you are naturally healthy mentally, physically, and emotionally, so radiance and intuition begin to form a shield of sorts that protects from negative external flows.

Now, when you go through a trauma, loss, or even just a mild event that caught you at a sensitive time, it's really common for a disharmonized emotional reaction to get lodged at a particular coordinate in your psyche as a glitch. When this glitch starts to calcify and catch more energy around it—think of a hurricane, anytime *any* kind of emotional trigger in your life hits that glitch or storm—you are going to respond the *same* way. Without some consciousness shaped around the habitual response, the glitch will try to complete the same magnetic pattern over and over throughout your life, whether or not the situations hold any similarity to each other or even to the original event that caused the glitch. Because we are ultimately computerized in our subconscious operating systems, input in a certain way will always run the same response program.

That pattern is mostly beyond your conscious awareness and is actually *looking for* and *creating* ways, situations, or people to allow it to run through its cycle. So it doesn't matter if your boss gives you a compliment or your spouse does that thing you hate—if the situation hits your glitch, the same response will arise. It could be like a perfect spring day or cyclone season, and you'd still be subconsciously preparing for a volcanic eruption.

One of the reasons it's so hard to break out of emotional patterning is that we have not, as humans, been given effective tools to demagnetize these glitches and therefore see them as such—which does make it seem insurmountable or hopeless. You might at least have developed the wherewithal to know that you *want* to change your emotional responses but have noticed that once some outside stimuli hits that glitch, it's *very* difficult to control your response.

An amazingly effective Kundalini Yoga meditation to fix magnetic subconscious self-destructive and commotional glitches is the Medical Meditation for Habituation.

In this meditation, you squeeze your back molars to create a new pattern in the hypothalamic rhythm of the central brain, which will increase the projective wattage of the pineal gland. Say what? Well, your habits and cravings all neurologically originate in the central brain. This meditation begins to reform those. What you will find through practice is that magnetic patterns that *were* looking for any and every avenue for self-destruction no longer need to complete themselves. And this is true for emotions as well as any other kind of habituation, such as cigarettes, heavy drinking, drugs, OCD habits, or relational sabotage.

The benefit of demagnetizing habitual tendencies, whether they are emotional or any other kind, is that you gain the freedom of choice. Human sovereignty is based on having enough energy to see that you have a choice in how you experience your own reality. This means you have command of your emotional spectrum and can use it as a tool instead of as a weapon. This is *so* empowering. When you feel empowered as a human being with your infinite capacity for creativity and immense compassion—you can and will have fulfillment. And when you experience fulfillment, naturally a wellspring of energy is tapped from which to *enjoy* your day, your relationship, your job, your children, and your life. And that overflow of natural human greatness is the core of yogic consciousness and practice.

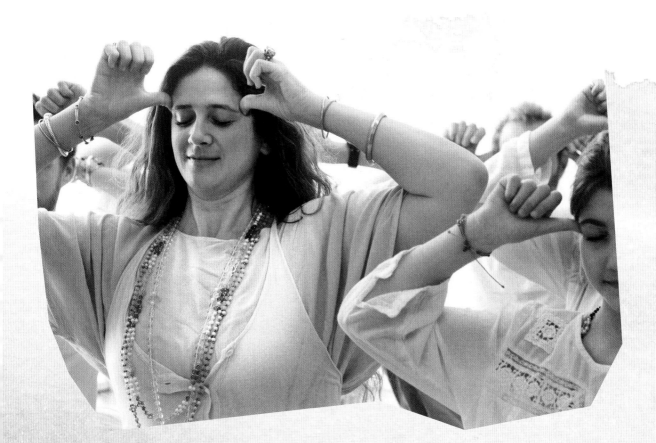

MEDICAL MEDITATION FOR HABITUATION

NOTE: This exercise is also called the Addiction Meditation.

POSTURE: Sit in easy pose. With both hands, curl your fingers into the pads of your hands— not into fists, just down so that the fingertips are resting right on top of the pads at the base of each finger. Leave your thumbs extended, and place them on your temples.

BREATH AND MANTRA: Breathe normally in and out. Mentally repeat the sounds *Sa-Ta-Na-Ma*. On each sound, press your back molars together.

You should feel something move underneath your thumbs. Keep going.

TIME: 3 to 11 minutes

TO END: Inhale, focus on the center of the forehead through closed eyes, set the frequency, exhale, and relax.

EMOTIONAL ENDOCRINOLOGY

I had the great gift to be in a small group of people with His Holiness the Dalai Lama in July 2015 around the time of his eightieth birthday. He was talking about how it's now the time on the planet when we start to scientifically understand the spectrum of emotions and how to command them. Something that the yogis of many lineages have understood is that you can get a powerful hold on your emotional experience through the *endocrine system*.

There's an actual physiological base to your emotions. There's a chemistry of the blood, a chemistry of the organ health, and a chemistry of the endocrine secretions that creates your emotional balance—or lack thereof. And it's all very subtle, because these are subtle systems in the physical body. However, your emotional mastery and acuity are *not* so subtle—they are real and profound.

When these secretions are out of balance, you feel irritable, cranky, aggressive. *But,* when the endocrine system is secreting properly, it is actually very difficult—I would say impossible—for you to act obnoxiously or moodily. When the endocrine system is in balance, *you* are in balance. You feel *good*. You have a connection to your infinite reality. You feel happy! If your glands are totally in the right balance for you and your body chemistry, there is no way you can be depressed. So it makes real and practical sense to have a baseline understanding of your endocrine system and the yogic tools to balance it at a moment's notice!

THE ENDOCRINE SYSTEM MADE EASY

Your endocrine system is collection of glands that secrete hormones. The major glands include the thyroid, parathyroid, hypothalamus, adrenals, pancreas, sex organs, and pineal, all headed up by the pituitary gland (also called the master gland), which controls all other glandular secretions. The job of the endocrine system is to trigger physiological processes, cellular growth, and emotional experiences through specifically coded hormonal releases.

If you experience anger, that's a distinct hormonal code running through your body via your circulatory system and bloodstream. If you are feeling depressed, that's another separate hormonal code. It's the same with happiness. And the more refined a name we have for a feeling, like *euphoria* versus *sublime,* or *pissed* versus *worked up,* the more specific the coded hormonal mixture.

This why you can talk to a therapist until you are blue in the face, but if you don't have techniques to command your endocrine system, you will still end up feeling depressed. And often, the repetition of trauma and unhappy events or situations through the retelling and reimagining of them, creates the exact same biochemical reaction and subconscious reality as the original event. And in some weird way the body gets used to or even addicted to these biochemical experiences.

The New Age woo-woo energy healer doesn't get a free pass either. Even if your shaman goes in and removes that block in your third chakra from your third past life, if your blood hormone levels don't get shifted, you end up with a hollow feeling and most likely a reinforced or reactivated hormonal pattern despite having spent a bunch of money. Then the trauma is often relived by talking about it or by re-creating it in a relationship or experience of reality. There is *no difference* between a real or imagined event to the subconscious mind and the body's subsequent biochemical reaction.

We all want a positive, fresh, balanced emotional experience, right? So that means we *have* to balance the glandular system on the regular. There are so many stimuli and patterns that throw it out of balance, so we do have to make a bit of an effort here. Luckily, this is so easy.

The Cold Shower practice I gave earlier is bar none the most effective glandular detox, balancer, and rejuvenator. And, if you do it consistently, it's a total antidote for depression. I can't say enough about cold showers. *But* if arctic temperatures at seven in the morning just aren't your cup of tea, you can also reset your glandular system with the Four-Stroke Breath for Balance.

The Four-Stroke Breath for Balance is powerful for glandular equilibrium because it balances out the pituitary gland. In yogic science, your pituitary gland is called the master gland. All of the other glands in your system take their direction from the pituitary. So your thyroid, parathyroid, pancreas, hypothalamus, adrenals, and sex glands (ovaries or testes) all change based on the secretions of the pituitary gland. This is the seat of endocrine system power and command! Your glands control the onset of emotional experience moment to moment. So you can completely alter your total experience of life by adjusting and balancing these secretions! Here's how it works.

FOUR-STROKE BREATH FOR BALANCE

NOTES: This technique will actually reset the hormonal coding response in your endocrine system and allow for the energy to move *past* the re-creation of suffering or unhappiness in your daily life. We have suffered enough, haven't we?

POSTURE: Sit in easy pose. Alternatively, you can do this at your desk, on the train or subway, in the car, or wherever you are.

EYES: Keep your eyes closed, gently focusing up and in at the brow point (or open and relaxed if you are in a public space).

BREATH: Inhale in four equal strokes through the nose. Exhale in four equal strokes through the nose. Continue.

TIME: 3 to 11 minutes

TO END: Inhale, hold the breath. Exhale and relax.

EMOTIONAL MIND

We're not wired to be depressed. Everything in our system is wired to be happy. But the first way that wiring goes off is through the habitual thought forms and the unconscious and subconscious mechanism of thought creation.

Our mind and our moods are our servants, but we think of them as our masters. The whole idea of understanding your infinite capacity for reality is that you have command over your mind and the thought choices you make. And, in turn, you will have command over your emotional spectrum.

Most people have one, just *one*, thought form that is making it nearly impossible for them to experience happiness and joy in this life. You might have a lot of negative thoughts. *I hate my life. Everyone is out to get me. My world is hopeless . . .* But most of the time, your thoughts are just various incarnations of your one primal negative thought—which could be something like *I'm worthless* or *I'm a failure* or *I'm scared*. All neurosis and subconscious thought forms come from the same place or similar places in your psyche. You pull one side of the string, and the rest comes tumbling out. It's the same string; it's all the same thought.

This thought form is running the way you think. It's throwing your glandular system off track. It's creating the glitch in your electromagnetic field. And it's disturbing your emotional well-being. It most certainly is affecting all of your intimate relationships in one way or another.

This is especially true about the whole idea of being depressed. There *is* biochemistry and a neurochemistry to depression, and I'll give some techniques for counteracting it. But depression is also a thought form that many modern people have ingrained in their minds.

You might have been someone who actually had a pretty easy childhood. But one moment, one day, one thought gets lodged in you in a certain way, and before you know it, you're depressed. So you start thinking about how depressed you are. And worrying about how depressed you are or might get.

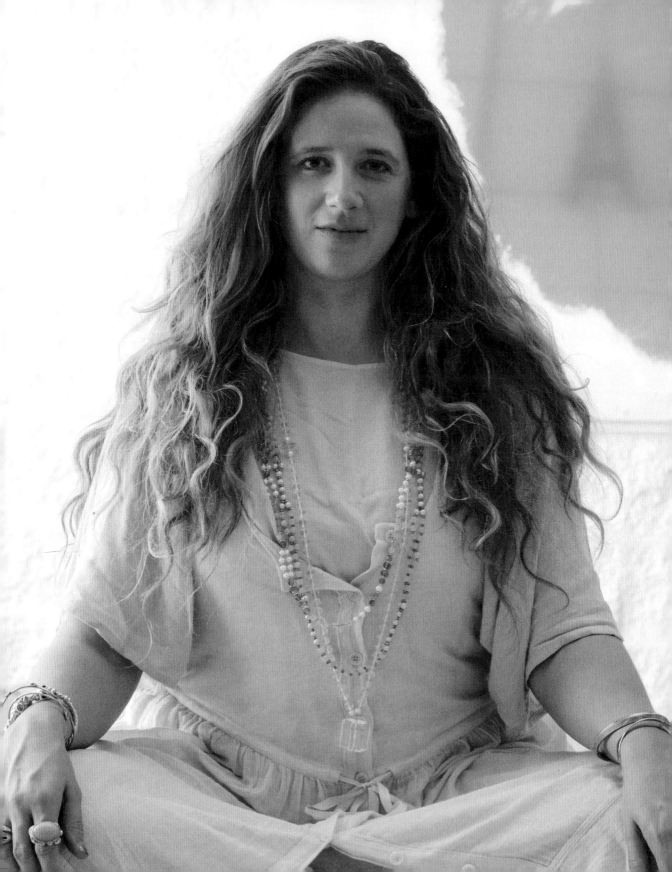

You start thinking, *Okay, I should go talk to someone because I'm really depressed.* So then you start talking about how depressed you are with whomever you are paying to talk about how depressed you are. And you're talking to all your friends about it too. So now you're just talking about depression . . . talking about depression . . . talking about depression. And re-creating the experience over and over in your system.

Finally, you get to someone who's going to *give* you something for your depression. And you figure you probably should take it because you're really depressed. I mean, you have convinced yourself and everyone around you that you're depressed. And when that doesn't work, they give you an anti-anxiety pill, and then they give you the antidepressant for the antidepressant. It can be a very detrimental and harrowing cycle.

And unfortunately the people who are prescribing many of these medications are being educated about the drugs' usefulness and side effects by twenty-five-year-old pharmaceutical reps over a nice sushi dinner. The pharmaceutical industry does *not* care about your true well-being, and the pharmaceutical rep is collecting a paycheck. In what I believe is a *global crisis* of anxiety, depression, and insomnia, we must start to educate ourselves on alternative ways to stabilize our emotional and chemical systems.

The more you say you *are* depressed, the deeper you start to believe that as your true emotional experience. And when that energy gets calcified, it's very hard to break out of! In neuropsychiatry it's called rumination—and it's *known* to calcify your trait into a state.

Rewiring thoughts and biochemical experience *can* be done using any of the breath exercises from this book or the Medical Meditation for Habituation. It's also a very effective thing to use a mantra for.

A short and small mantra that is great for redirecting your thoughts is *Sat Nam* or *Sa-Ta-Na-Ma*. *Sat* (sounds like the *u* in *rut*) is a sound current that replicates the sound of the Universe. *Nam* (sounds like the *o* in *tom*) refers to form. When you mentally or vocally repeat *Sat Nam*, you are sending a sound signal both to your cognitive brain and to your endocrine system to bring your form or finite self into the infinite of the Universe. So it's a great tool for changing the looped pattern of your normal thinking. The word *mantra* refers to "mind" plus "vibration" or "wave" and is a directive to your complex and amazing mind.

SAT NAM MEDITATION

You can practice Sat Nam in a meditative fashion by sitting in easy pose, focusing closed eyes on your brow point, and mentally reciting *Sat* on the inhale and *Nam* on the exhale. What's great is that this is another practice you can do anywhere at any time. Just inhale *Sat* and exhale *Nam* and watch the results.

One thing is certain—a human system that has deep breath, deep oxygenation, and glandular balance actually cannot hold lower states of experience like depression and anxiety for very long if at all. They can pass by for a moment, but they can't take hold and create a long-term systematic experience-and-reexperience cycle. Your breath, including the depth of your breath, is yours to practice and experience, and it costs nothing. Breathing deeply and consciously will only benefit you in ways you can't even imagine at this moment.

THE MIND AS TIME-SPACE MACHINE

For those who have experienced a trauma that triggered the original depression, the mind was given to you as the greatest gift—it is truly a time-space machine. If you use it correctly, you can actually traverse time and space,

MEDITATION FOR REMOVING HAUNTING THOUGHTS

POSTURE: This practice can be done anywhere.

EYES: Close the eyes nine-tenths and focus on the tip of the nose.

BREATH AND MANTRA: Breathe normally and direct the mind in the following manner:

1. Mentally vibrate *Wah* as you focus on the right eye. Mentally vibrate *Hey* as you focus on the left eye. And mentally vibrate *Guru* as you focus on the tip of the nose.

2. Bring up the bad memory. Remember the encounter or incident that happened to you.

3. Mentally say, *Wahe Guru,* as in number 1.

4. Visualize and personify the actual feeling of the bad memory.

5. Again repeat, *Wahe Guru,* as in number 1.

6. Reverse the roles in the encounter you are remembering. Become the other person, and experience that perspective.

7. Again repeat, *Wahe Guru,* as in number 1.

8. Forgive the other person, and forgive yourself.

9. Repeat, *Wahe Guru,* as in number 1.

10. Let go of the incident, and release it into the Universe.

TO END: Inhale and hold the breath. Exhale and relax.

back to the moment of trauma wherever it is in your time continuum and psychomagnetic field, and actually change and heal the memory. Which means, in your life, you have the instant power to no longer operate from that trauma prison—you are not limited by the bad or challenging things that have happened to you or around you. In fact, you can use them to have victory.

I encourage you to experiment with this power of your mind. Try the exercise given on the previous page.

When I am feeling any emotional sluggishness, I also like this physical way for getting that heaviness out of my ten bodies.

JUMPING OUT OF DEPRESSION

Jump with your arms reaching up toward the ceiling for one minute. Breathe deeply through the nose as you do it.

Every time you jump off the ground—every time you try to pull your body weight off the ground—the body associates that with "I have to get lighter," so the brain and all the ten bodies associate that activity with getting lighter. When this occurs, you're starting to dump the negativity. Every body has to get lighter, so not just the physical body but also whatever's murky in your subtle body, mental bodies. Everything has to get lighter.

SELF-PSYCHOLOGY

In this modern age, with the acceleration of human evolution and the pressure of technology, we're all working with an increased demand on some level in the body and the brain. I'd like to introduce you to the power of *self-psychology*.

PRACTICE FOR SELF-PSYCHOLOGY

On your smartphone, make a recording of how great, talented, and amazing you are for at least three minutes. Listen to it once a day for a week and see what happens!

Self-psychology is a simple modality Yogi Bhajan taught through which you can bypass years and years of individual therapy, a lot of money, and recapitulation of the original trauma over and over—and heal yourself with some simple self-practice and intention.

When your glands are in the right balance, your mind becomes more and more free of looping thoughts and you begin to reset your brain chemistry, and then your natural ability to self-adjust into happiness happens at a moment's notice. That's the power of these practices and the possibility of human potential at this time on the planet. Just ask yourself, what would happen if we had a society filled with emotionally stable, courageous, generous, and integrated human beings? Everything, including our economic systems, families, and societal norms, would upgrade in the light of a new human dignity. It's a profound vision to behold, and your personal day-to-day command of mind and body systems is an integral part of this vision. Plus, it will simply make you feel better, so you will do better, think better, and be better.

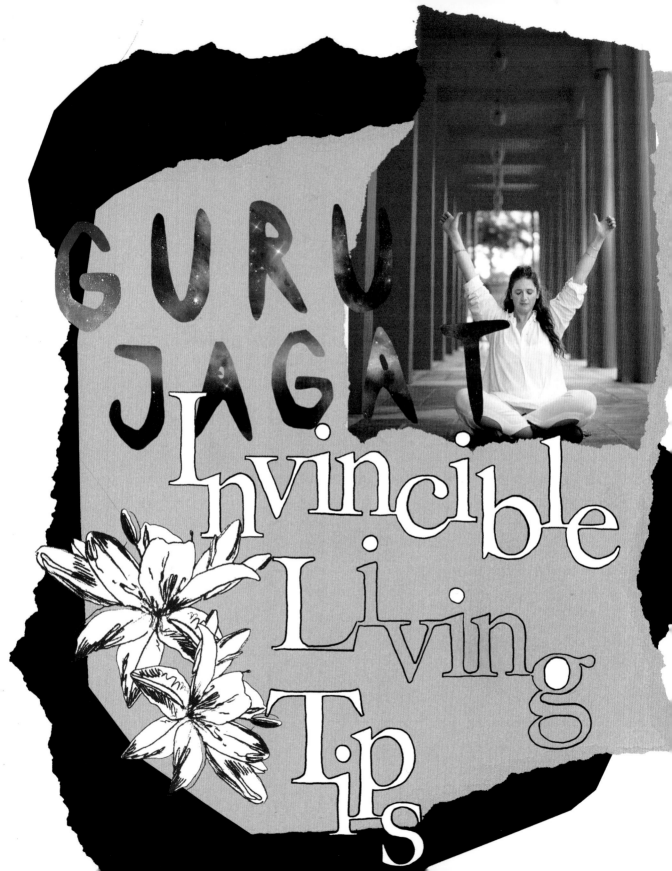

Wake-Up Set

Yogi Bhajan, January 30, 1985

This short, electric set is enough to tune me up for the whole day! I love how it's also good to do this kriya in bed as a way to help you get up and get going.

1. **Stretch Pose.** Come onto your back. Stretch the legs straight and together, and lift them 6 inches off the ground. Raise the head, neck, and shoulders 6 inches off the ground and point the hands toward the toes. Hold the position with a Breath of Fire, eyes fixed on the toes. Hold for 1 to 3 minutes. To end, inhale, pull root lock, exhale, and relax.

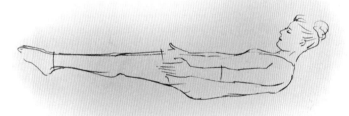

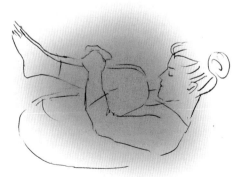

2. **Nose to Knees.** Immediately bring the knees into the chest and clasp them there with the arms. Bring the head up so that the nose comes between the knees (or as close as you can get it there). Breath of Fire. Hold for 1 to 3 minutes. To end, inhale, pull root lock, and concentrate the energy on the brow point, exhale, and relax. Then roll on the spine and come up to easy pose.

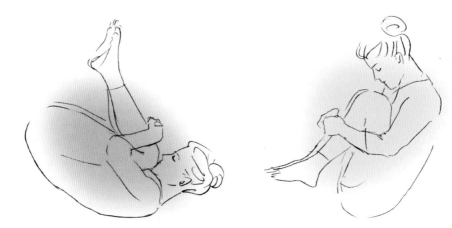

3. Ego Eradicator. Sitting in easy pose, curl the fingertips to the top pads of the hands, leaving thumbs straight. Raise the arms to 60 degrees with thumbs either pointed toward each other or up toward the sky. Hold the position with a Breath of Fire for 1 to 3 minutes. To end, inhale and hold breath, raising the arms overhead so that the thumbs magnetically touch. Stretch the spine tall. Exhale and slowly sweep the arms down, energizing your auric field. Press the fingers into the earth. Relax and feel the light around you as you meditate on your illumined being.

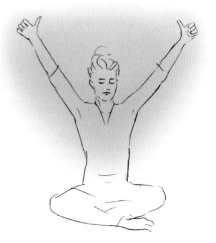

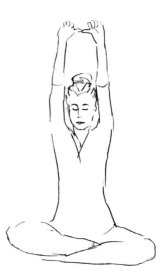

When I'm feeling out of balance, I adjust the chakras. Chakras are direct psycho-emotional energy centers for how we experience the world.

Eighth Chakra
Aura
Projection of Shimmering Personality, Protection from External Negativity

Seventh Chakra
Fontanel Center
Divinity, Royalty, Clarity, Radiance, Universality, Love, Reverence

Sixth Chakra
Third-Eye Brow Point
Intuition, Perception, Deep Sight, Focus, Answers

Fifth Chakra
Throat
Inner Truth, Self-Expression, Grace, Creative Collaboration

Fourth Chakra
Heart Plexus
Love, Compassion, Peace, Harmony, Healing

Third Chakra
Navel Point
Power, Will, Effectiveness, Get Things Done

Second Chakra
Sex Organs
Sex, Self-Esteem, Creativity, Emotional Balance, Relaxation

First Chakra
Sacrum
Money, Security, Home, Physical Strength and Wellness

A fast way to align the chakras is to adjust the navel point with exercises like Stretch Pose or Breath of Fire. Once the navel point is set, all of the other chakras start spinning at their highest and healthiest frequency.

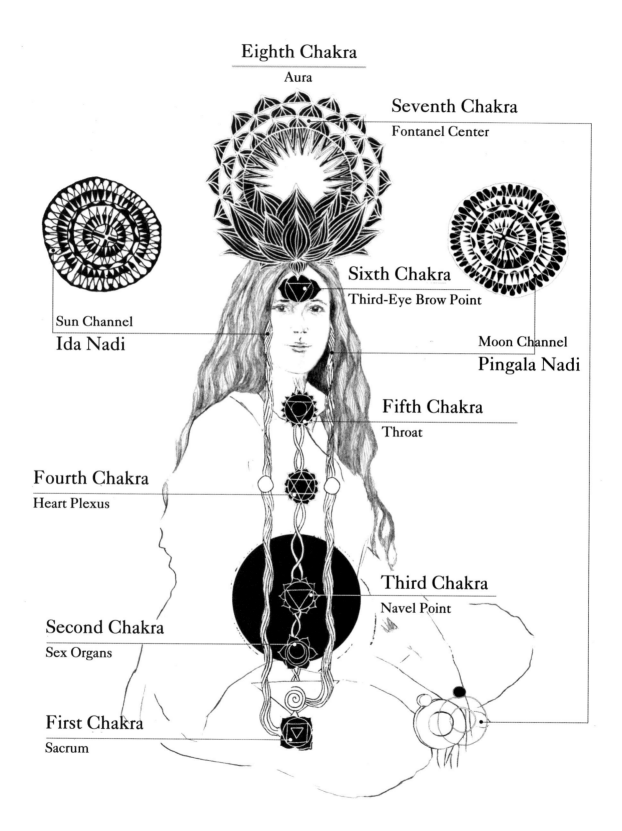

Eighth Chakra
Aura

Seventh Chakra
Fontanel Center

Sixth Chakra
Third-Eye Brow Point

Sun Channel
Ida Nadi

Moon Channel
Pingala Nadi

Fifth Chakra
Throat

Fourth Chakra
Heart Plexus

Third Chakra
Navel Point

Second Chakra
Sex Organs

First Chakra
Sacrum

Surya Kriya

I use this set for whenever I need to kick a cold or energize myself for a big day. It activates the solar energy, which purifies the body and gives you the vibrancy to light up a room!

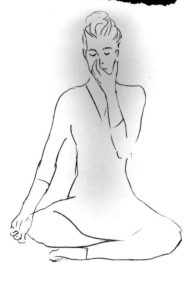

1. Right-Nostril Breath. Sit in easy pose and rest the right hand on the knee, index finger and thumb tips touching. Take the left hand and block off the left nostril with the thumb. Keep the other fingers of the left hand spread and pointing straight. Breathe long, deep, and powerful through the right nostril for 3 to 5 minutes. Inhale, exhale, and relax.

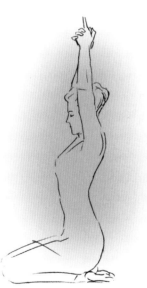

2. Sat Kriya. Sit on the heels. Bring the arms overhead, steeple the index fingers and interlace the rest. Women cross the left thumb over right; men do the opposite.

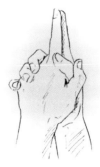

Rhythmically chant *Sat Nam,* pulling in on the navel as you powerfully chant *Sat* and releasing it as you chant *Nam.* Continue for 3 minutes. Inhale, hold the breath, pull root lock, and imagine energy radiating from the navel and circulating through the body. Exhale and relax.

Take a few moments to integrate. Then repeat the exercise for another 3 minutes. To end, inhale, pull root lock, and draw all the prana to the top of the fingertips. Exhale and relax.

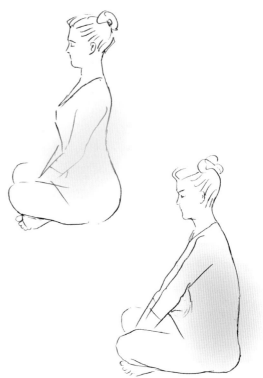

3. Spinal Flex. Sitting in easy pose, grasp the shins with both hands. Inhale as you flex the upper spine forward, opening up the chest. Exhale as you let the lower spine flex backward. Keep the head level. Flex the spine 108 times, mentally chanting *Sat* at the third eye as you inhale and mentally chanting *Nam* on the exhale. To end, inhale to a straight spine, pull root lock, exhale, and relax.

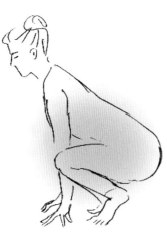

4. Frog Pose. Come up to standing. Place the heels of the feet together and point the toes apart so that the feet are forming a V shape. Now, lower your body into a deep squat so that the heels come off the ground. Place the tips of the fingers on the ground to steady yourself.

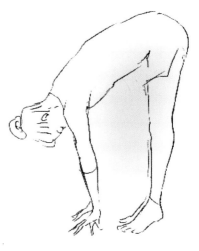

Inhale and lift the buttocks up, letting the forehead come toward the knees. Exhale, lower the buttocks, and lift the head and chest. Keep the fingers on the ground the whole time, and try to keep the heels lifted and together. Repeat with deep breaths 26 times. To end, inhale up to stretch the back of the legs. Then exhale and relax down onto the heels.

5. Neck Turns. Sitting on the heels, place the hands on the thighs. With a straight spine, inhale, mentally chanting *Sat* at the third eye as you turn the head to the left. Exhale, mentally chanting *Nam* as you turn your head to the right. Continue for 3 minutes. To end, inhale with your head centered, pull root lock, exhale, and relax.

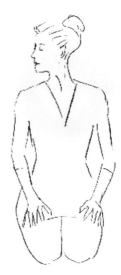

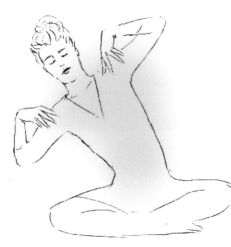

6. Spinal Bend. Sitting in easy pose, bring the arms up parallel to the ground and grasp the shoulders, fingers in front and thumbs in back. Inhale and bend to the left; exhale and bend to the right. Continue this stretching with deep breaths for 3 minutes. Then inhale straight, pull root lock, exhale, and relax.

7. Meditate. Stay in easy pose and relax your hands on the knees, index finger and thumb tips touching. Keep your spine straight and relax, pull gently on the navel, and keep a light root lock. Watch the flow of breath and meditate on the brow point. On the inhale, listen to a silent *Sat*. On the exhale, listen to a silent *Nam*. Continue for 6 minutes or more.

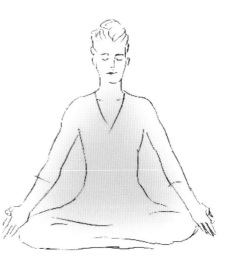

The Glandular System

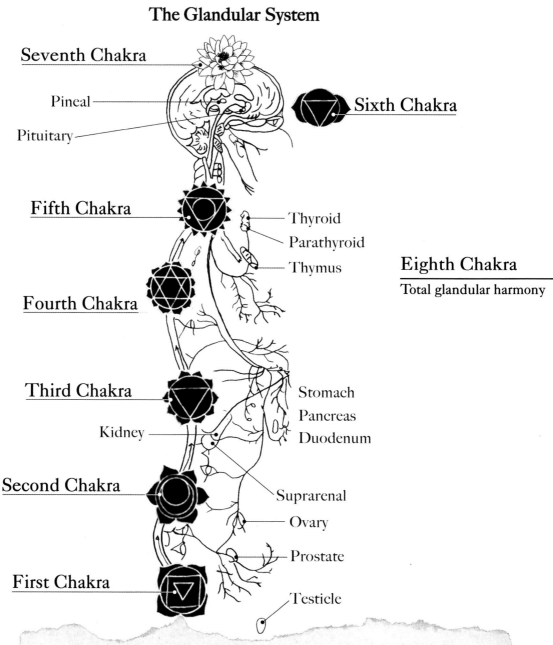

Seventh Chakra

Pineal

Pituitary

Sixth Chakra

Fifth Chakra

Thyroid

Parathyroid

Thymus

Eighth Chakra

Total glandular harmony

Fourth Chakra

Third Chakra

Stomach

Pancreas

Duodenum

Kidney

Second Chakra

Suprarenal

Ovary

Prostate

First Chakra

Testicle

It's amazing to me how our physical and energetic bodies match up. Every gland in the biological body directly corresponds to a subtle wheel of energy in the auric body. The wattage and brightness of the Crown Chakra depends on the health and suppleness of the pineal gland. The Sixth Chakra, also esoterically called the Third Eye, perceives more deeply and intuitively based on the secretions of the pituitary gland. You can see here the tangible interconnectedness of your chakras and physical systems of the body.

Kundalini Yoga: Let the Liver Live

Yogi Bhajan, January 30, 1985

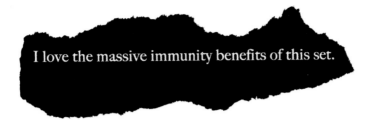

I love the massive immunity benefits of this set.

1. Right Leg Lift. Lie down on your left side. Supporting your head with your left hand, elbow resting on the ground. Lift the right leg as high as possible and hold the toes, or knee, or what you can, with your right hand. Keep both legs straight. Begin Breath of Fire and hold for 4 minutes. Inhale, pull root lock, exhale, and relax.

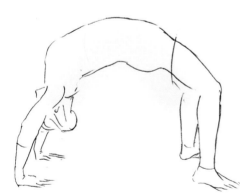

2. Wheel Pose. Lie on your back and bend your knees, bringing feet flat on the floor a comfortable distance from the buttocks. Take the arms over your head and set the palms on the ground above your shoulders, fingers pointed toward the feet. Push yourself into an elegant arch. In this posture, breathe alternately through the nose and then the mouth. Inhale, exhale nose. Inhale, exhale mouth. Continue for 4 minutes. Inhale, hold breath, pull root lock, exhale, and relax.

Modification: If you can't push yourself into a wheel pose, it's no big deal. Simply bend your knees and bring your feet flat on the floor a comfortable distance from the buttocks. Bring the arms down by your sides, palms against the floor. Then push the hips up as high as you can into a bridge pose.

3. Left Leg Lift. Repeat exercise #1 with Breath of Fire through the mouth for 2 minutes.

4. Deep Stretch. Come up to standing. Bring feet 18 to 24 inches apart. Bend down and stretch your hands through your legs as far as possible. Keep the head down, and try to touch the floor. Hold for 1 minute with normal breathing, Then, staying in position, roll the tongue and do Breath of Fire through the rolled tongue for 3 minutes.

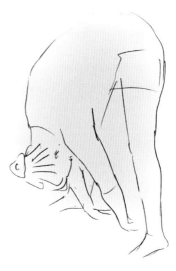

5. Left Leg Lift. Repeat exercise #1 with Cannon Breath. Inhale through the mouth and exhale through the mouth with an extremely powerful, explosive breath. Continue for 30 seconds.

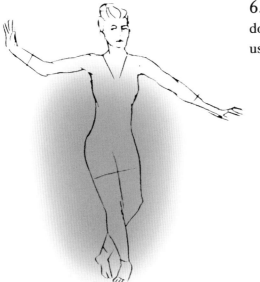

6. Stand/Sit. Stand up and sit down on the floor 52 times without using the hands to support you.

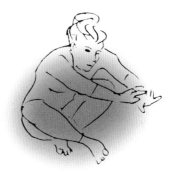

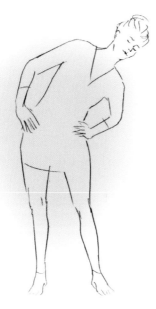

7. Torso Roll. Stand and bring your legs to a comfortably wide stance. Lean your torso one direction and swing it around to make large circles with your torso around the hips in one direction. Continue for 2 to 7 minutes.

Top of Head

Activates the crown chakra

Brow Point on Third Eye

Stimulates the pituitary gland and opens up intuition

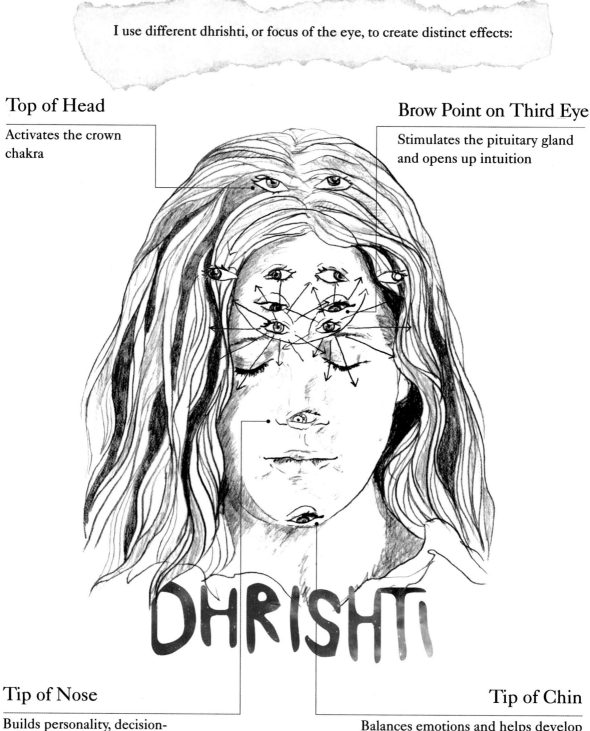

DHRISHTI

Tip of Nose

Builds personality, decision-making clarity, and forethought by strengthening the frontal lobe of the brain

Tip of Chin

Balances emotions and helps develop grace and nobility

Weight Loss Set

Yogi Bhajan, August 31, 1995

Anytime I detox, I add this short kriya to my daily practice for the week. I suggest you start this kriya by holding each position for 1 to 3 minutes. Then, if you are inspired, gradually and gently work your way up to the maximum time.

1. Camel Pose. Kneel with your knees about two fists apart. Press your hips forward and, supporting your lower back with your hands, arch backward. Open the heart, throat, and chest. If you feel good here, stay. If you have more flexibility, release the hands onto your ankles. Stay open and graceful and breathe normally.
Maximum time: 11 minutes

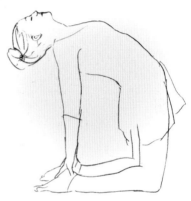

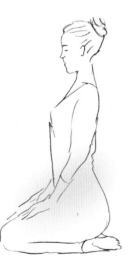

2. Rock Pose. Slowly come out of camel pose and come sitting on your heels. Place your hands on your thighs, sit straight, and focus at the brow point. Breathe meditatively.
Maximum time: 11 minutes

3. Baby Pose. From rock pose, bring your forehead to the ground in front of your knees. Bring your arms beside you, palms facing up. Breathe and relax.
Maximum time: 11 minutes

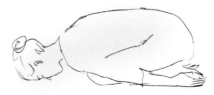

NEXT LEVEL EYE CARE

I brighten dark circles, calm puffiness, and hydrate the thin skin around my eyes using organic ghee—a.k.a. clarified butter. An advanced practice of this secret Ayurvedic beauty art includes taking an eye-cup of melted ghee and washing the entire eyeball with the oil. It makes the whites of your eyes brighter and the pupil more radiant.

DEEP HEALTHY HAIR

This is my favorite yogic hair-care trick: Take 1 to 4 tablespoons of almond oil and mix in a few drops of sandalwood oil. Apply to the scalp and massage to stimulate the roots. Take a shower to shampoo the excess oil out of the hair and wait till the locks have fully dried before combing. It's a surefire method for strong, shining, sweetly scented tresses.

ABSOLUTE SKIN

Washing the face with the coldest water possible is a powerful stimulant for collagen production and cellular radiance! It's why I'm known to seek out the most glacial temperatures for my face rinse. If you decide to take this practice on, try following with a bit of almond oil and sandalwood to seal in the moisture. Almond oil mimics our body's natural moisture serum and sandalwood tones the skin and prevents wrinkles.

NADIS

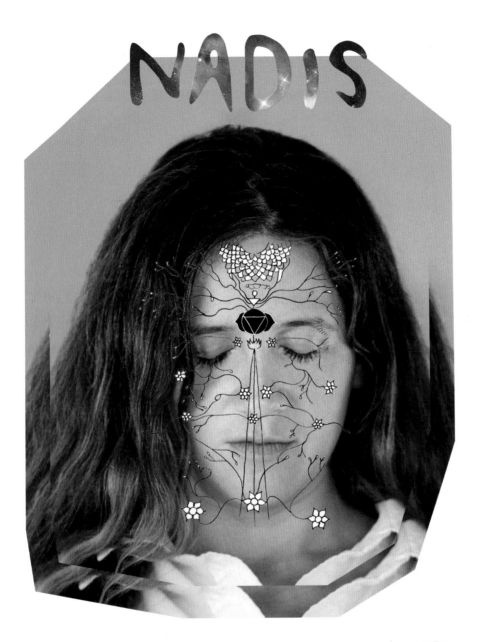

Another way I tune myself throughout the day is by noticing the quality of my energy and adjusting the appropriate *nadi*. Nadis are circuits of pranic energy and the three main currents are the *ida*, *pingala*, and *Shushmana*.

IDA—The *ida nadi* directs calming, lunar energy. If I want to relax or cool down, I concentrate the breath through the left nostril, where the *ida* channel ends.

PINGALA—The *pingala nadi* moves energizing, solar energy. If I need to focus or wake up, I breathe through the right nostril.

SHUSHMANA—When I'm looking for meditative clarity and neutrality, I focus on breathing through both nostrils to activate the *Shushmana*, the central *nadi*.

The Hand of the Cosmos

Conch   Totality, Flow of Life
Third Eye   Intuition, Wisdom

Mercury   Communication
Emerald   Prosperity
Lilac   Sweetness

Sun   Life
Ruby   Sun
Rose   Romance

Saturn   Purity, Knowledge, Piety
Blue Sapphire   Saturn
Iris   Purity

Jupiter   Knowledge, Grace, Wealth
Yellow Sapphire   Jupiter
Lotus   Purity

Mars   Lord of Victory, Happiness
Id   Binding Factor of Life: Soul, Body
   & Mind

Coral (reddish)   Mars
Marigold   Victory, Rejoicing
Mound of Venus   Love
Venus   Love
Tulip   Creative Power, Opens Up Progress,
   Expansion
Diamond   Love

Moon Mound   Mind, Thoughts, Strategy,
   Planning, Fantasy, Fears
Pearl   Communication
Moon   Pearl
Lily   Communication
Ganesha   Success
Hanuman   Lord of Strength

Kundalini Snake   Central Power of the
   Universe, Existence

Heart Line   Kindness, Compassion, Caring
Head Line   Strength of Direction of the Mind
Life Line   Length of Life Span, Breath of Years
Fate Line   Challenges to Be Met
Relationships   Social, Sexual, Sensual
   Interaction

7 Chakras   Seven Energy Centers
7th Chakra   The Tenth Gate

Wealth Arrow   Prosperity

Three Rings of Destiny   We don't exist without
   these: Life (Courage),
   Love (Prosperity), and
   Happiness (Compassion)

One of the things I love about Kundalini Yoga is how fully it understands the infinite nature of the human. This map, originally created by Yogi Bhajan, shows how much massive cosmic power we hold just within the palm of our hand!

The Hand of the Cosmos

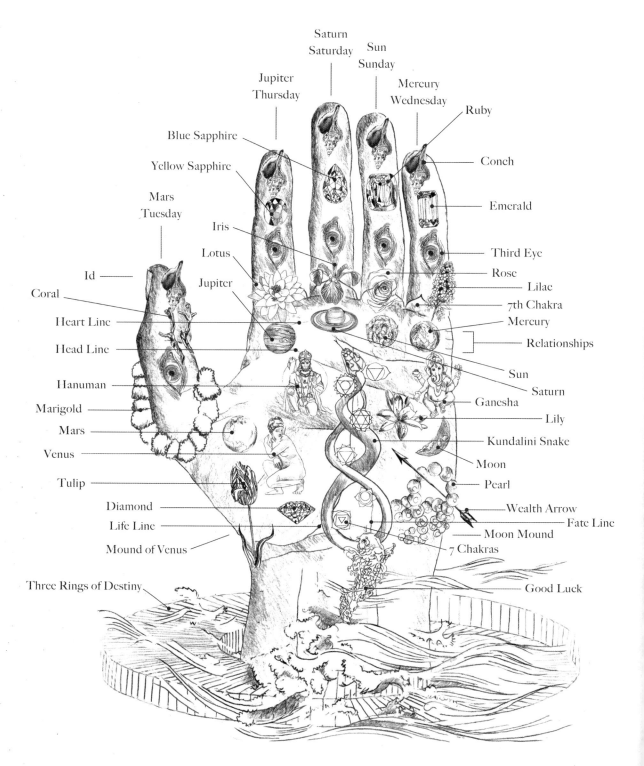

Only you can crown yourself!

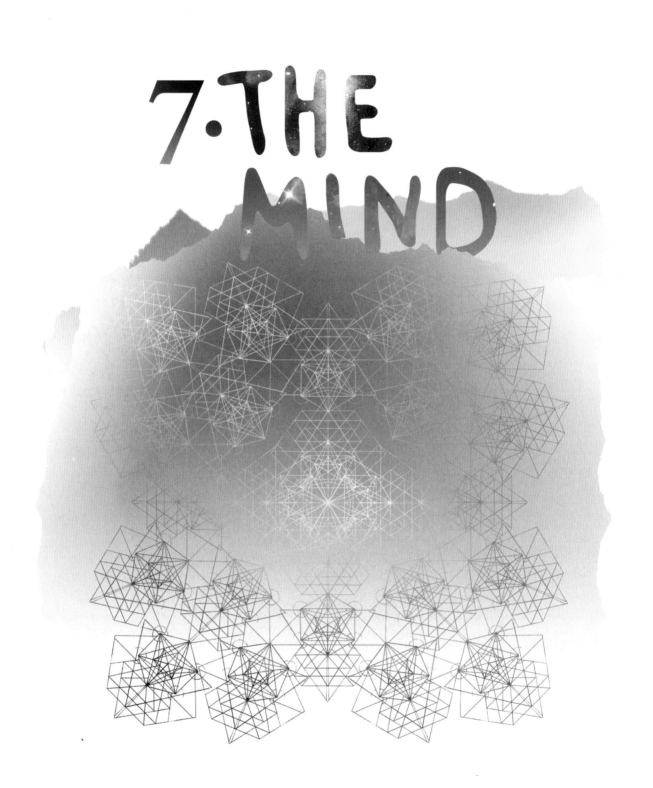

7.THE MIND

As I have said, your mind is the greatest gift you've ever been given. It traverses time and goes beyond space. Given the right direction from the heart, it coordinates the rest of your ten bodies into action. It has the immensity of thought and allows you to cognize experience. So the mind is an incredible gift, but it's also kind of like a toddler.

Sometimes toddlers like to get into places where they're not supposed to be and make toys of things that are not supposed to be toys—like kitchen knives! So your toddler is running around with a kitchen knife—not good. You chase after the kid, exchange the knife for a feather duster, and let the running begin again. That's almost exactly the way you need to treat your mind, and meditation becomes a tool to do so. The purpose of meditation in the Kundalini technology is not to slow the mind down, particularly, or even to rein in its massive energy and power. Just to give it constructive tools and direction and allow for that to create new pathways of thought and experience.

Just like you wouldn't give your toddler the steering wheel of a car and say, "Go for it," it's not too wise to let your mind take the steering wheel of your life. Which is what an untrained mind will try to do. The untrained mind is a headstrong kid that's always trying to take the wheel and derail you into some version of self-destructiveness.

We've allowed the collective and personal mind's untrained destructiveness to take over all of our media, politics, economy—really all of society. And we don't have societal training in the West, particularly, to train the mind on a daily basis, whether through nature, meditation, or any contemplative practice.

One of the major problems with an untrained mind is that it will not allow you to command the time and space of this lifetime. When you leave the mind untrained, it will make you feel as if you are barreling out of control and will give you the corresponding anxiety and fear responses.

You have only so much time and so much space to live this life, and it is all so very precious. Rather than let you waste this life on the teeter-totter of a toddler's whim, I want to give you some tools to navigate your mind toward success and satisfaction.

TWO THOUSAND CHANNELS

Your mind needs to be trained to be able to know and recognize the *vast* spectrum of thoughts and experiences that you can participate in or choose in *every moment*.

I'll give you the equation that Yogi Bhajan taught us. In every blink of an eye your mind releases *a thousand* thought forms.

1,000 thought forms / 1 blink of the eye

In the thousand thought forms, each thought has a *positive* and *negative* ionic pole. So now we have two thousand choices per every blink of the eye.

$$(1,000 \text{ thought forms x 2 ionic poles}) / 1 \text{ blink of the eye}$$

We're only ever really vibrating one thought at a time, which means that there are *1,999* other thoughts that we leave behind and therefore dump into the subconscious mind, which has finite storage capacity.

$$[(1,000 \text{ thought forms x 2 ionic poles}) / 1 \text{ blink of the eye}] - 1 = 1,999$$

So if you are in a situation where you feel limited, or you feel lost, you're suffering, you're scared—or fill in the blank with the plethora of human misery—if you're stuck in some experience that is not your highest quality, your highest vibration, your highest directive of experience, then you actually have *1,999* other experiences in every single moment that you could choose from. This is liberating to at least become aware of!

Life is a choose-your-own-adventure experience. If you don't like the channel you are on, you can change it! Now, in order to do this, you have to know that there are other channels. Then you have to know that there is a remote control. You have to know where the remote control is, and *then* you have to know how to operate the remote control! Learning the controls of your mind is not *that* difficult.

In order to even *know* that there are choices, you need to have *energy, health,* and *vitality.* Most people are so energetically depressed (different but related to emotional, psychotherapeutically identified depression), they are stuck in their particular rut of misery and can't fathom the idea of having the possibility of another channel. So the notion of four or five channels, and especially 1,999 channels, is way out of conceptual range because you need to have energy and clarity to even see the rest of the spectrum. And once you can see the possibilities, even if it's just *one* additional possibility, then you need to have enough energy, wherewithal, and awareness to change the channel.

We normally think of energy in terms of caffeine boosts, sugar highs, marathons, and other sorts of hyper activities. This is energy, sure, but it's not

Your mind needs to be trained to be able to know and recognize the vast spectrum of thoughts and experiences that you can participate in or choose in every moment.

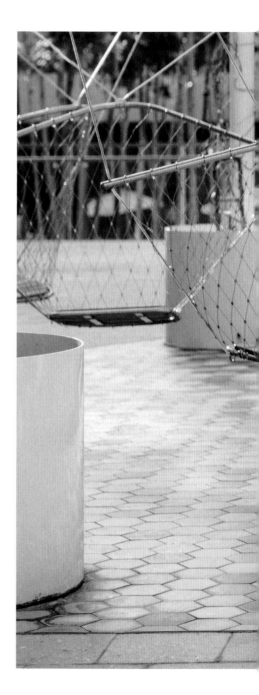

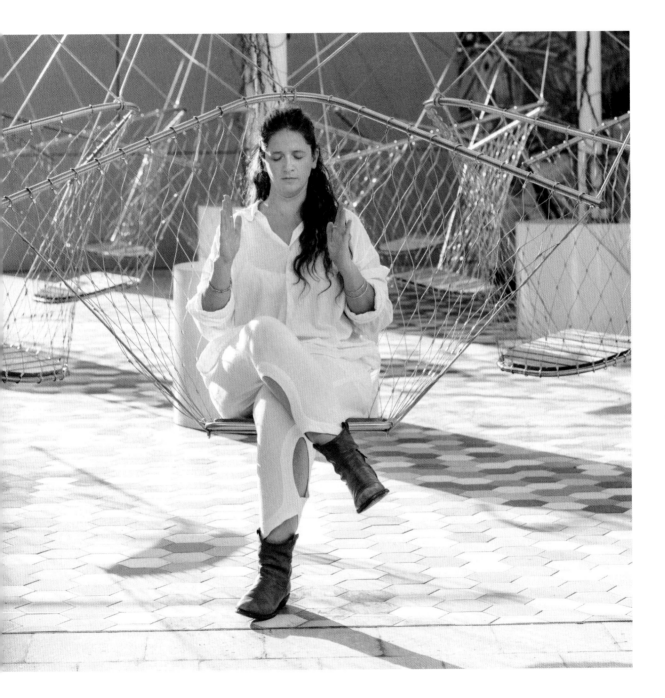

the kind of energy needed to toggle between the thousands of options you have. In reality, we know that caffeine and sugar are ultimately depleting. And the energy it takes to kickbox, hit the weight room, or run a marathon is actually just the very surface of the kind of energy I am referring to.

Energy is a kind of wattage in the system, which, again, isn't hyper. A hyper system is one that is fritzing out, so it's actually using the energy inefficiently. A system with *wattage* is a clean, cool, running battery. It's noiseless. But it can take you from 0 to 320 in 0.09 seconds if you need. And it's nuanced. It doesn't have just two speeds. It can drive the vehicle of your human being at 60 mph just as easily as it can drive at 60.25 mph. Energy, real energy, is powerful but also very *intelligent*. This is what you need in order to shift the channels of your mind.

One of the best ways to generate more energy in the system is with the breath, as I've been saying in many different ways. *Prana*, this word I've been using a lot, is an ancient yogic term for "energy," and it exists everywhere in the known Universe. Prana even exists in the black vacuum of space. Prana can be taken in through the eyes and through the pores. Eating fresh foods is a great way to get more prana. However, the easiest way for most people to metabolize prana, and lots of it, is through the breath!

Ancient yogis actually called structured breathing practices pranayams because they knew that breathing was just a way to get more prana into the system. One of my favorite pranayams is the Aerobic Capacity and Efficiency Breath. I give it on the opposite page, and it's a very simple but effective way to amp the wattage of your physiological and energetic bodies.

MEANING OF *MANTRA*

Mantras, or sound codes, are also a very effective method for re-tracking the mind toward better thoughts. The word *mantra* tends to scare off people if they're not interested in any dogmatic belief system. And I get it—we've had

AEROBIC CAPACITY AND EFFICIENCY BREATH

POSTURE: Sit in easy pose and grasp your knees with your hands.

EYES: Keep your eyes closed, gently focusing up and in at the brow point.

BREATH: Inhale and hold your breath. Now flex your spine back and forth, using your hands on your knees to create leverage. Flex at a smooth, rapid pace. When you can't hold the breath anymore, bring your spine to neutral and exhale. Inhale here, hold the breath, exhale, and begin again.

TIME: 3 to 5 minutes

TO END: Sit straight, inhale, exhale, and relax.

enough of those. It can seem intimidating, complicated, religious, or spiritual. But mantras, as I've stated, are codes and nothing more than vibrations that affect your neurology or your glandular system in a certain way.

Actually, *mantra* means "wave of the mind" or "mind direction":

MAN—man, mind, or mental being

TRA—vibration; directional vibration

So a mantra is a mental wave—*any* kind of mental wave. But a chanted mantra is simply a sound that directs the flow of the thoughts.

And the way we use mantras in Kundalini Yoga technology is just a specific mental wave that directs the flow of the thought to something *higher* than the lowest common denominator. *Sat Nam,* for example, is a high-caliber sound that connects you with your most authentic beingness. We're trying to train the mind to pick up higher vibrational thought waves rather than your mind's lowest common denominator—*Same shit, different day,* or your particular version of a negative or habitual thought.

There is an alchemical process that happens from the sound. And we're just scratching the surface of what the technology of sound is and how it works in Western science. MRIs are a sound technology. A study at McGill University measured the brain chemistry of people before they made a sound or sang a song as well as afterward. The brain chemistry of people after singing or chanting was much more serotonin and dopamine rich! So we're starting to get some research around the same sound science that as yogis we have known for thousands of years, which is exciting and very important.

Jappa, the repetition of highly tuned sounds, has a kind of alchemical process discovered in yogic science through repetitive practice. The yogic term for this alchemical process is *tappa.* Mantra is the sound, jappa is the repetition, and tappa is the alchemical process that takes the mind from negative and self-defeating thoughts to something more positive and clarifying.

For the most part, the repetition, the jappa, of your thoughts is the repetition of a subconscious mantra that is connected to self-hate, self-doubt, or self-failure mechanisms. And that's what's getting repeated over and over. When we introduce into the system a repetition, a jappa, of a more stable and self-supporting sound current, then everything starts to change.

There may seem to be a lot of yogic or spiritual jargon involved in certain mantras, but in reality it is a science. No one is interested in indoctrination. We all want activation into our highest self. You can use the science of the sound to begin to clear the finite storage space of the subconscious mind. When you do this, it creates a space for more creativity and flow of actual experience in life, as opposed to past and future yo-yo thought games, or what are called mental intrigues.

MANTRAS

Since every thought is a mantra, I check in regularly with the subconscious mantra in my head. If I don't like the direction, I supplement it with a more uplifting, creative mantra from yoga.

Sat Nam—Truth is my identity

Sa Ta Na Ma—Infinity, life, death, rebirth

Wahe Guru—Incredible enlightenment

I am bountiful, blissful, and beautiful!

Ek Ong Kar, Sat Nam, Siri, Wahe Guru—There is one creative pulse, truth is its name, it is great, beyond all description.

Ong Namo Guru Dev Namo—I bow and link myself to the creative force inside me and beyond me, I bow and link myself to the divine teacher that is inside me and above me.

Har—Power and divinity

Victory!

When the going gets tough or whenever I feel like a little elevation, I chant a yogic mantra out loud. Chanting out loud uses the tip of the tongue to stimulate the eighty-four meridians on the roof of the mouth in a particular code to activate healthy brain chemistry and emotional balance.

STORAGE UNITS, HOARDERS, AND THE SUBCONSCIOUS MIND

Now, when you don't process the other 1,999 thoughts you've had, where do you think they go? They unfortunately don't just fly off into the Universe. The *one* thought you have chosen broadcasts and creates reality momentarily. The additional 1,999 options get stored in the subconscious mind.

One of the *only* things that we have in us that is finite, besides the physical form, is the subconscious mind. For the most part, we are infinite creatures. Yes, our physical bodies are finite, but our souls are infinite. Our subtle body, radiant body, auric body, arcline, and pranic body are all infinite. Even the powers of the mind are infinite, and the mind is actually a tool to be *able* to navigate in this infinity. But the subconscious mind itself is *finite*.

There's some crazy, yogic calculation for how large the subconscious mind is. Yogi Bhajan said that it's some 8 million miles north, 8 million miles south, 8 million miles east, and 8 million miles west—so, it's big. But eventually *finite*. So it can and *does* get full! And any kind of stress tick, weird behavior, or neurotic thought pattern is always a symptom of an overflowing subconscious mind. But the subconscious mind can be cleaned through the process of meditation and sound technologies.

A good pop culture reference for the subconscious mind is the TV show *Hoarders*. I love that show. I play it whenever I'm cleaning my house to scare myself into throwing stuff away.

There's one episode I saw where this woman, this really sweet woman, had filled up all *fifteen* storage units of the local storage facility. Year after year, she kept buying and filling and buying and filling more and more storage units until there were no more left.

I'll never forget this one part of the episode. The woman was so sweet, and she was just pleading for more storage units. The owners of the place were so uncomfortable, because there weren't any more! It was really heartbreaking.

And that's a great metaphor for the subconscious mind. It's finite. You can only fill it with so much. Once it gets full, you start to get crazy, anxious, depressed; you start to have nightmares, insomnia, and suffer through all kinds of epidemics. Then these stress epidemics that you're suffering under because of your full subconscious start to leak out into your unconscious and conscious mind and, as a result, become more and more of your waking *reality*.

It's a law of being in the human form on this planet that the subconscious mind *has* to be cleaned. Just like you take a shower to clean your body, and you clean your house, anything that is finite must be cleaned. Because when we don't clean the subconscious, we get psychic, emotional, and mental buildup. But when we *do* clean these finite arenas, our home, our body, and our mind are that much more beautiful. They sparkle. And then there is room for something more magical and creative to come in.

So this meditative work is—in my belief—a requirement, but many of us were not really taught any kind of mechanism for cleaning the subconscious mind other than possibly some prayer practice. And prayer is powerful, especially when it helps us to connect to something more infinite inside of us. But generally we have no secular practice to clean out the subconscious mind.

When you start to bring more energy into the system, say with a pranayam or any other practice that I've given in this book, the mind will automatically start to clean itself. You will naturally begin to dump subconscious thoughts. For this reason, don't be alarmed if you feel negative or something bizarre comes up during or after meditation. This is *always* a good sign that you are releasing some old garbage from the storage bins.

A lot of people don't like meditating. As soon as they sit down, the mind starts releasing, which is a *healthy* thing, but it scares some people off. The only advice I can give is to keep going! Don't back off. Living in a house stuffed to the gills with old newspapers is way worse than the kind of courage you have to muster to take out the trash. Don't identify with the thoughts—just let them filter out. Meditating will become easier with continued practice. And you just have to remember that you *always* feel better after taking a shower or cleaning your room. Always.

TRAUMA BROADCAST AND THE TIME-SPACE MACHINE

When you don't clean the subconscious mind, you end up with what is called a trauma broadcast, which is kind of like the *Peanuts* character Pigpen. You're carrying around a lot more dirt than you need or want to, but you've collected it and now it's with you and playing a part in how people see you and feel you and concurrently how you see the world.

Your mind is not subject to time and space, but when properly trained, the mind is useful to move through time and space. You can project into the future, to some imagined possibility or even a *real* situation that you know is going to happen. You can also take yourself back to when you were four, eating pasta at your grandparents' summer home. Close your eyes and remember a time from earlier. You can take yourself back there, can't you? And you can re-create all the emotional biochemistry from that instance too. So it actually starts to *feel* the same. This should show you how easily the mind can traverse the time-space spectrum and direct your experience of reality at any given moment.

Oftentimes we are unconsciously projecting trauma or some traumatic event that haunts us into the world on a daily basis, long after the event occurred. This then becomes like a satellite broadcast or a WiFi signal. And, even more often, this trauma broadcast has been with us for many incarnations, in our various lifetimes and familial lineages. The study of epigenetics is finding fascinating things about how these traumas actually pass from generation to generation on the cellular level.

So these trauma or fear broadcasts can be heavy and can carry through generations or lifetimes. *I'll never be loved. Success is threatening to my safety. Everything bad happens to me.* What happens is that you are projecting this into a thought wave or beam through time and space. It's in your "now," but it's also projecting into your past *and* projecting into your future. Layman's quantum theory maintains that past, present, and future all exist simultaneously. So as we subconsciously identify and broadcast into the future from the past or from now, a trauma pattern starts to accumulate energy and create reality. Then when we catch up to it in the future, we say, "Look, there it goes again—I knew it." The trauma broadcast becomes a self-fulfilling prophecy.

What we have the opportunity to do through Kundalini Yoga and meditation is actually *move* our mind to different situations in the past and rewrite them. Go into the past, surround a moment of trauma pain or grief, heal it, rewrite it, and recalibrate it.

REWINDING THE TAPE

A powerful practice for redirecting the energy broadcast of your mind is called the Daily Rewind Exercise. The exercise was given to me by my teacher Harijiwan and is traditionally a nighttime practice, to prepare the subconscious and unconscious minds before sleep. However, the practice can be done at any time provided you are in a space where you have a couple of minutes of quiet. This is not the kind of practice that you can do on the subway or while driving. It needs your focus and attention.

It is typically done on a daily basis to rewrite any of the trip-ups you encountered during that day. But you can also rewind the tape as far back as you want to rewrite all the traumas, failures, and missteps you've experienced along the way. This practice is tremendously healing for all wounds obtained in any part of your life.

DAILY REWIND EXERCISE

DIRECTIONS:

1. With your head on the pillow, mentally scan through your day. It's called rewinding the tape. Just rewind and watch your day from beginning to end.

2. When you get to a part of the day when you didn't act in your highest integrity, you missed a crucial piece of information that led to a mistake, or you encountered a situation that triggered a trauma experience for you, stop the tape. Rewind and watch that part again.

3. How could you have responded differently? What did you miss? How would you rather experience that moment in time?

4. Now rewind again, and this time write over the tape. Rewrite the experience to be one that honors the reality of the circumstances but also allows you to feel that you acted with utmost intelligence, wherewithal, and personal strength.

5. Then rewind one last time and watch the tape with the newly inserted scene in which you are secure, clear, and confident. Now that moment is an empowerment to you, even if the real-world consequences of it are still the same.

6. Keep going until you feel complete.

Do it sooner rather than later so you don't get stuck in that thought form for more than just this lifetime. Clear the trauma, the nervousness, the anxiety, the depression, and the self-criticism. Rewrite it through higher intelligence. Then all of a sudden your projection into the future—and your projection for this very second—will become *intrinsically* different.

CHANGE YOUR PERSPECTIVE

In the current Technology Age, we are being forced to build a mind that can more easily compute the clearing of its own neuroses, subsequent fears, and other malfunctions.

Meditation is like muscle training for the mind. Its results are more valuable than gold.

Here's what meditation will really do. So you've got a thousand thought forms, two options for each; you've got an overflowing subconscious storage unit partially full from trauma broadcasts in this lifetime and others. A meditative mind will give you the ability to change *perspectives*.

Most of our lives are caught in one perspective, or imprisoned in a limited perspective of whatever's happening in the short term, the context of our daily lives. We often feel very stuck because we are caught in one, maybe two, perspectives of life. But our mind, just our mind *itself*, has *eighty-four* facets. What that means is that there are eighty-four perspectives that can be toggled through in any respective moment. That's very powerful.

ONE-MINUTE BREATH

POSTURE: Sit in easy pose, hands in gyan mudra.

EYES: Keep your eyes closed, gently focusing up and in at the brow point.

BREATH: Inhale very slowly and deeply for 20 seconds. Hold the breath in for 20 seconds. Exhale slowly for 20 seconds. Continue this breath. Very slowly, very deeply and in exact proportion. If you can't inhale, hold, and exhale for the full 20 seconds, start with 12 seconds and then work your way to 14, 16, and then 20. To measure the count, use the mantra *Sa-Ta-Na-Ma.*

TIME: 3 to 11 minutes (up to 31 minutes with practice)

TO END: Inhale, exhale, and relax.

In yoga these days, there's a major fixation on these fancy physical yoga poses and all the competitiveness and injury thereof. In the whole canon of yogic practices and teachings, these advanced postures, the whole reason for the pretzel-shaped one-armed handstands, is to give you a *physical metaphor* for a change in mental and emotional perspective. The handstand is just a physical symbol for how you can put your body into a shape that is going to turn the whole situation upside down, a change in *perspective.*

Our job as advanced humans is to be able to change perspective as needed, to move between varied input sources and certain parts of our faculties as modern humans. We need to be able to do that mentally, emotionally, and in all sorts of other ways. So thinking that getting your body into some x-y-z posture is the be-all and end-all of yoga is a total illusion. It's just a tool to be able to get your mind to see from an x-y-z perspective.

And you can get that from asana or a physical experience, but you can also get that from meditation. In Kundalini Yoga, we use both to create the change in perspective even more rapidly. The physical energy is filtered through the meditative mind and the sound current.

More and more people are flocking to some sort of meditative practice. These meditation practices are essentially self-hypnosis and give you the ability to not be hypnotized by the external comings and goings of life. This also allows you to navigate time and space in a way that does not project suffering or pollution to the people and environment around you. This then means you have the power to change the channel, clean up, heal yourself deeply, and have fruitful and positive perspectives on your life!

Being a *human* means that you are a *hue* (light) and you are now. You are the light of now. You are not only a collection of bones, organs, ligaments, and muscles or hopes, fears, desires, trauma, and jealousy. You are made of light, sound, prana, and energy. This understanding will instantaneously put everything in perspective.

A really powerful meditation to activate the eighty-four facets of your brain is the One-Minute Breath given on page 168. It heals the totality of the brain and gives you access to your complete cognitive intelligence. This is a lifelong practice, and you can start small and steadily build on your breath capacity. If you can't do the breath for the whole minute, just do what you can, take any adjustments you need, and work up to the full time.

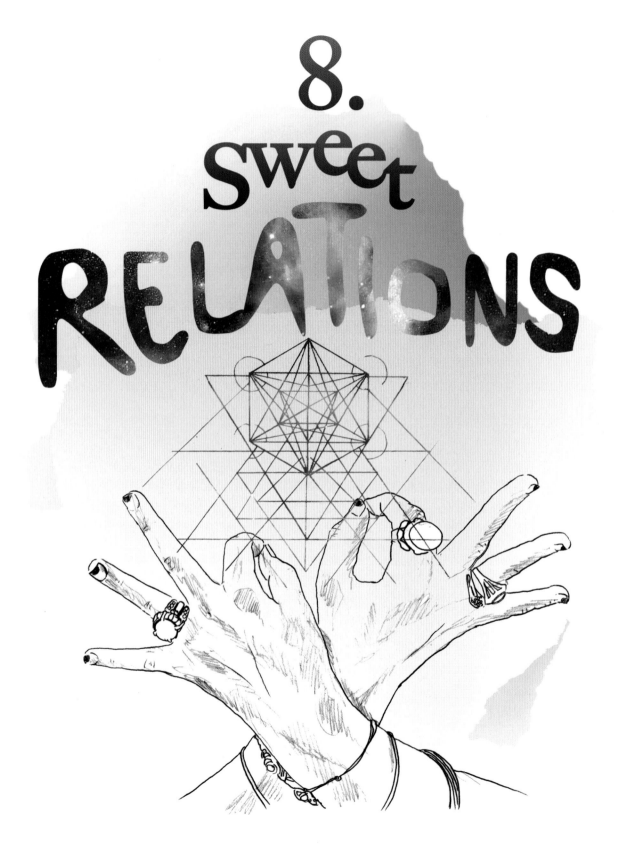

8.
Sweet
RELATIONS

Relationship is truly the greatest yoga. Yoga means the union of opposites or mastery of polarity. And a good relationship should be an expression of that in all of its aspects. It is also the greatest yoga because it tends to be the most *confrontational* yoga; it offers you the greatest and most intense possibilities for evolution and personal transformation at a rapid pace. Because relationships of any kind are microcosmic and macrocosmic simultaneously, they are one of the biggest pieces to a satisfying life.

But in today's new age of virtual realities, instantaneously deleted communications, social media gratification as a toxic mimic of intimacy, and dating apps, there's now a wider spectrum of what relationship looks like. From casual dating and serious courtships, to lifelong marriages and conscious uncoupling, there's room for all kinds of relational experiences, which makes it more difficult to get the most out of our relationships, whether they last twenty-four hours or twenty-five years. Because what's possible in relationships today is constantly changing, we need the skills to handle the multilayered complexities of the new relational playing field. Mastering the tools necessary to get the most out of any relationship is one of the most valuable investments you can make. And I'll give you one hint—the way you get the most out of any relational experience is about giving what you want to receive.

These yogic relational agility tools give you the ability to relate consciously and pleasurably across the entire range of the relational spectrum, which can add excitement and authenticity to any relationship, regardless of its length or intensity.

WOMEN DATING

Most women want to be in some sort of a relationship. It's our nature. Women are wired for relating, community, and family, so when you're not in an intimate relationship, most likely you're on some level looking for one. And that usually means some version of dating or socializing.

Conscious dating requires you to activate and use your *innate sensitivity.* Whenever you meet someone, as a woman you have a native intuitive wisdom about how that interaction will play out. If you listen to your intuition and train yourself to do so more and more, you can save yourself a lot of time and heartbreak, or at least you can consciously experience something in relationship rather than feel victim to it.

Your intuition works fast, anywhere from three to nine seconds. So you know within *three seconds* of the beginning of your date—or, actually, within three seconds of *seeing him or her on screen*—what that date is going to tend to be like or at least if it's worth your time to figure it out. You know if the date is going to be interesting, fun, sexy, boring, okay, or whatever. Intuitively you can know exactly what it's going to be like. The human sensitivity level is getting quantumly more active. Back in the day, even five years ago, you might not have had this faculty or didn't know how to get in touch with it, but there also wasn't the velocity of a computerized age to contend with. And with this sensitivity, you can make a decision about spending time and energy going out with this person or not.

YOGIC ENERGY EQUATION

X Amount of Energy + X Amount of Time = Your Day / Life

What I will say here is that this is *not* a question of morality or being judgmental. The binary device of the mind is always judging—that's part of its faculties. So it's a real New Age poison to think that you can stop that inherent mechanism from running the information through a bifurcating, binary, black-and-white, program. Once that is done, which again happens within seconds, then there is the more qualitative discernment of intuition, which we are taught *not* to listen to from a very young age.

That being said, even if you feel or intuit that this may not be the guy or gal for you in the long run, or that something is happening that may not be your highest spiritual blah blah, that doesn't mean you don't choose to experience whatever it is. This skill and faculty isn't about not having fun or experimenting with whatever you need or really just want to experience. However, the more you are conscious of your intuition, the more likely you are to find clarity while cutting through your own patterns of self-deception, which leads to a more fulfilling and honest experience, relationship, or date.

If you are having trouble activating your innate sensitivity, a good way to tap into it is to begin to train yourself to follow the intuitive voice and stop second-guessing yourself. Start doing it with something more practical like how to dress yourself in the morning or how to find your way somewhere following innate sense of direction. Second-guessing yourself is one of the fastest ways to cut your connection to your intuition. Your intuition can always be refined, but you first need to develop a relationship with it. So start by training yourself to listen to at least the first impulse.

First thought, best thought. It's actually a powerfully deep teaching. You're not just training your mind for the first thought, but you are training your whole mind-body system for the first complete thought that creates clarity and a deeper "breath" in you—physically, emotionally, or mentally.

Now, these are very simplified ways of starting to connect with complex processes of intuitive power in your system. And there are a lot of other factors to determine and cultivate your intuition. Another way to connect is to ask yourself the question and then sit for a couple of minutes focusing on *Sat* on the inhale and *Nam* on the exhale. This is a good way to clear the mind's layers of clutter that are addicted to patterns that may not be serving your highest good.

Other yogi tricks to increasing intuition are really focusing the eyes at the brow point during any yoga exercise, meditation, or pranayama—unless the instructor or directions specifically tell you otherwise. When you focus at the brow point, the cross of the ocular nerve stimulates the pituitary gland. Your intuition and the power of your sixth chakra—the *Ajna*—are based on the amount and rhythm of the secretions of your pituitary gland. As you breathe slowly and open up your sixth chakra, you will develop a more subtle awareness of your intuition.

Try sitting for a moment after a strong breath practice and sense the energy circulating and gathering around you. After a really powerful breath exercise, your cells are clean and activated. They are awake and sensitive and can read the energy field with striking precision. Sitting for a minute after a pranayama or meditative practice will help to develop this connection and intelligence. This quiet moment can find you in the middle of a tough decision and help direct the right action. When I practice this personally, I just go in the direction of the highest amount of energy, which is pretty obvious in many ways when you train yourself daily to pay attention.

DATING SPECTRUM

If every date you go on leaves you feeling dissatisfied, it's time to look at the lowest common denominator of those dates. You. If you are looking for a partner and you continuously find partners who are similar in some ways but *not* in the way that you want, look at the projection that you are putting out there.

Relationships and dating can be subtle. Men (and women) respond to *energy flows,* oftentimes without even knowing it. If you keep encountering people you consider to be slimy or who don't treat you the way you want, you are in some way broadcasting old subconscious baggage or self-fulfilling prophecy that is attracting them. This is not about you feeling bad about yourself or using it to reinforce your self-loathing. Simply consider it a point of reference to get honest with yourself.

On the flip side of the coin, a date of a really high caliber, or simply with someone who's a lot of fun, will respond to the kind of *radiance* you project outwardly to them. Not just a physical radiance but an energetic radiance.

It's important to really take note that men are *not* attracted to the size of your jeans only. That's complete propaganda designed to disempower you. Quality men are attracted to *energy.* So if you are in a space of openness—if your heart is open, if your breath is open, if your subtleness is open, and if you are broadcasting radiance—you are going to start to become *very* attractive to the kind of men you most likely want to be spending time with.

When you begin to practice any of these techniques, one of the more amazing things that happens is that you clean and clear your aura, which is the energy house you live your life in, and therefore you naturally will start to radiate more. These practices also affect your arcline, which is best shown in Renaissance art as the angelic halo above people's heads. This is actually a phenomenon of your more subtle self. I cover more about arclines in the next chapter, "Sex Is Science," but in the meantime, here is a really powerful practice for increasing your radiance.

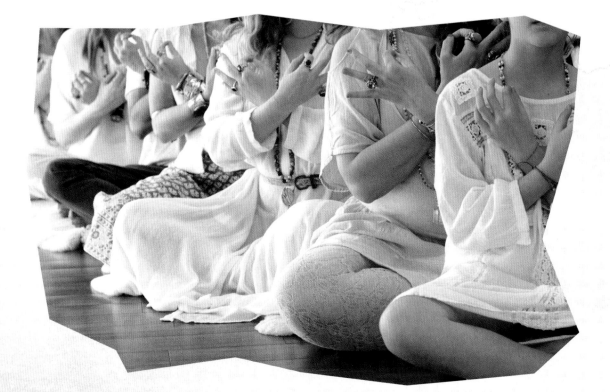

CROSS-HEARTED KIRTAN KRIYA

POSTURE: Sit in easy pose. Cross your wrists in front of your heart. The palms are facing the body and also slightly up.

EYES: Focus your eyes on the tip of your nose.

BREATH AND MANTRA: Breathe normally. Out loud, say each syllable of the mantra *Sa-Ta-Na-Ma* as you alternate touching each finger to the thumb. So on *Sa*, you touch the tip of your index finger to your thumb. On *Ta* you touch your middle finger with your thumb. On *Na* you touch your ring finger. On *Ma*, the pinky finger. Do it monotone or check out the melody on RA MA TV.

TIME: 3 to 11 minutes

TO END: Inhale, exhale, and relax.

LOOKING TO GET SERIOUS

If you're in the market for deeper partnership, there are a few dating tools that will help you develop the connection you want.

At an unconscious, biological level, men are looking and yearning for devotion and support for their purpose on the planet from the woman they choose to spend time with. This is an energy that so many modern women are either devoid of or refuse to embody on some level. *Devotion* in the post-feminist age has a bad connotation. It's been misunderstood that it means giving up your personal power in some way. And while the concept of devotion *does* mean service, it *does not* mean servant. Devotion means you come with a level of self-confidence, self-containment, and self-reliance that allows you to support your love's purpose or mission. That's true devotion. And if you can begin to practice that, you will start to attract someone of a high caliber, one worthy of your devotion, exactly the kind of person you're looking for, and exactly the kind of human you deserve if you're practicing giving in this way. What *caliber* really means is that you attract a love who is reliable, steady, deep, wise, and ready.

We want to go into a potential relationship with openness and experimentation and for some kind of exchange or experience that isn't just transactional. But the "what have you done for me lately?" consciousness is very programmed into the way we function in relating.

When you start fixating on a specific type of person, which is normally what we are doing when we go after first-impression physical attraction—automatically a transactional relationship is created. Either consciously or unconsciously, you think that type is going to do something for you—raise you socially, give you a certain kind of life, be great in bed . . . whatever. Standards are healthy, but many of our concepts around attraction, what attracts us initially and what keeps us attracted, are transact-ory, When relationship becomes primarily transactional, then it always fails. *But* if it is resurrect-ory, meaning open and fresh and looking to revitalize and rejuvenate each other, discover something new together, creating love and curiosity between each other, then it will always win!

> *If your caliber is trans-act-ory . . . you will meet failure after failure, after failure, after failure. And if your caliber is resurrectory . . . you shall succeed, and you shall succeed, and you shall succeed, and you shall succeed, or you can be in between, you understand?*
>
> —YOGI BHAJAN

Since all relationships are a dance of polarity, even in same-sex relationships, these archetypal tendencies and energies run through each partner. In order to keep things hot, alive, electric, and working, both people have to acknowledge their respective opposites and recognize how these opposites work to create the good tension and healthy friction in relating. There's some strange post-feminist notion that we are looking for a mate that is like us in some ways, and I can tell you that the more a partner is *not* like you, the more possibility there is for sustained chemistry, which is always the long-term relationship quandary.

Now, you can actually work to polarize a relationship after there've been too many same-same activities—grocery shopping, movie watching, parenting, etc. These functionary or mindless activities are important and can also be made hot, but mostly they don't create attraction.

It's also important to note that often you are most attracted to people who hold some sort of magnetic pattern that is *not* good for you particularly. This subconscious recognition is often experienced as heavy physical attraction.

Our first impressions are frequently related to our parents and subconscious stuff, rather than what's going to move us or what's going to change us. Now, whether you want to take that on or not is your choice. But I think what it highlights is that what we're attracted to at first sight isn't really what's going to take us to the transformation that relationship holds the potential for.

A way to know if you've found a solid, reliable partner is to look at the quality of his stance, particularly his legs. Yogi Bhajan always recommended that women discern the viability of their partners by looking at them from the feet to legs up.

How do they stand? It's not about how great looking their legs are but about how exactly they position themselves in relationship to the earth. Are they floating? Are they rigid? Is there energy there at all? It seems simple, but this embodiment will tell you a lot about how the man shows up in all of his activities, relationships, and work. It's a bio-communication that broadcasts the energetic profile of his character.

See if you can, for yourself, perceive the archetype of a man just by decoding the body language. It's a metaphoric and intuitive practice. But through the practice you will start to bring more subtlety into your choicefulness and thus deeper satisfaction.

WOMEN IN RELATIONSHIPS

Now, when you get into the space of an actual relationship, or if you're currently in a relationship, one of the most important things you can do is look at the relationship like you look at other practices in your life such as exercise, eating well, or anything else that requires you to show up in a certain way.

When trouble's a-brewing, I hear a lot of women complaining about their male partners and what is and isn't happening. He's this, he's that. He's lazy, he's an asshole, he didn't fix what you asked him to, and so on. The thing about this dynamic is—and I say this to women all the time—if you're having a problem in a relationship, you've got to look at *yourself*. Because a woman's intention and energy holds the *caliber* of the relationship.

Now, that doesn't mean you are or aren't the boss in the relationship. It simply means that you *hold the energetic level* for your partner to elevate and inspire into. If you are having a problem with your partner, look at what kind of energy you are putting out into the space of your relating. Is it elevating? Is it positive? On the surface, you could be hip enough to know not to complain or nag outwardly about or to your partner, but underneath the surface you could still be sabotaging the relationship with a nonverbal stream of expletives.

Most women are still detoxifying a lot of anger from an age of violence and adversarialism between the sexes. As we detox our own personal anger, we must recognize that our lingering anger, while directed at our partners consciously or subconsciously, often has nothing to do with them. Believe it or not, men want so badly to meet women where they are and even—*gasp*—to make them happy. It's a terribly unproductive belief that men are not evolving as fast as women are. They are trying as hard as they can, but it is up to women to hold open an elevated vision for them. Blaming men for lingering anger between the sexes keeps worthy men out of this space of actualization. And more important, out of your space. This belief is like a man repellant.

And if you are in a same-sex relationship, remember all of these concepts relate in one way or another, particularly ways to consciously work with power struggles and subconscious subterfuge in relationships.

There are many really good yogic ways to offset some of this anger in a relationship, ways that leave both you and your partner with a sense of release and relaxation, and a kind of cleansed energy.

The best way to work with a partner, especially a man, is to use *subtle signs.* No one wants to feel antagonized by the human being who they expect, and deeply need, to be their best friend. We know that disagreements happen, as do lapses in communication, which can turn into arguments. But rather than give in to the hypnotic pattern of relational aggression, it is possible for us to work to the level of clarity and patience to work on a deeper and far more effective level. These are the yogic arts of true change and discourse.

SUBTLE SIGNS

Anytime you talk to your partner, *particularly* male partners, start by looking at the area of the forehead right between the eyebrows. Esoterically we call this the third eye, but it also is the location of the pituitary gland. If you pulse and project your message—a positive one, please—into the area of his pituitary gland, you will actually make *a lot* of progress in getting what you want! This is the space where your partner will truly receive your message and have the ability to metabolize and even act on it! This is such a sweet way to start creating depth in your communication. And it is an especially good technique if you want your partner to do something—like some kind of chore. This replaces nagging. And it isn't manipulation; it's more like subtle positive reinforcement.

Even if you are not face-to-face with your partner, you can beam over a message into their third eye. The incredible thing is, your partner will receive the message as if it were *their* idea. You are able to then insert your intuition and special feminine intuitive clarity into the decision-making or situation, and their ego stays intact. This is *healthy!* When your partner does pick up the message or the nuance, make sure you overtly exclaim that it is a good idea or you really like where they are going or taking you. This will help them make better decisions in the future.

You can even just pulse a mantra like *Victory* into the third eye to help your partner elevate their own consciousness, something you both want. You may be surprised, if you pay attention, how much negative rhetoric you are thinking about your partner during the course of the day. So to turn around even just a bit of that into positive energetic reinforcement and good elevating thoughts will make an impact on him. Again—your partner *wants* to make you happy.

REAL RESPONSIBILITY

While women have to maintain the energetic caliber of the relationship, this doesn't mean men get a free pass. Without question, there are definitely situations that call for leaving a relationship.

Taking responsibility means we honor men and ourselves and know that when something is off, if there is bad air, *we* have the capacity to clear it on multiple levels. Men are much more simple and direct in how they look at the world. If they tell you they want an apple, they want an apple. If we say we want an apple, we may want an apple but . . . *Oh, I don't feel like an apple anymore. Are there oranges or bananas? Are they organic?* If you're in a relationship with a man, you're in a fairly simple situation. When it comes to relationships, men who are in relationship with women are the ones who have it much harder! But, as very complex beings, women have the capacity to maneuver the relational scene and do it gracefully and intelligently for the upliftment and health of all involved.

This relationship topic is vast and really could fill the pages of this whole book, but if you take one thing from this conversation, understand that as women, we directly create the future, literally, through our own bodies in childbirth. So when we are graceful and strong, compassionate and clear, we can *create* the energy of relationships that are hot, kind, and fulfilling to all parties involved.

If you are looking for a quick meditation for grace under fire—just say to yourself, "I am bountiful, blissful, and beautiful." Say it over and over until at least some small part of you believes it or remembers it. Doing this will strengthen the heart, clear insecurity, strengthen the clarity and projection of the mind, and generally support and allow for your true female essence to live and breathe.

MEN IN DATING

Through the maze of relational complexities, one thing that's very certain is that men are totally different from women in how they operate in the realm of dating, loving, and relating.

Regardless of sexual orientation, the male and female bodies contain certain standpoints of biochemical behavioral and preferential attitudes toward the major themes of life. I am going to be talking a lot about predominantly heterosexual men in this section, but it's important to understand that all relationships and attraction are about the laws of polarity, which exist beyond gender and sexual orientation.

I know you're unique as a man. I don't want to change you, and I'm not going to give you some female-driven advice on how to be more sensitive or do more yoga or meditation. What I am going to do is give you some tools to honor your nature and to navigate the relational experience more efficiently and intelligently.

Dating should be a place that allows experience and growth of more of your elementary self. I like and use the word *masculinity,* but it is such a tricky word, especially in the current discussion of gender identity and multi-layered sexual orientation. I live in Muscle Beach, and I'm certainly not talking about some caricature or concept of what being manly looks like. It also doesn't mean the media's or music industry's creation of pimps or players. It's not a *GQ* Man of the Year self-concept either. It has virtually nothing to with gender identification either. Masculinity means that as man if that's where you identify, you feel and therefore act strong, dependable, creative, and empowered—there's a connection to a deeper meaning of life and death than to shallow sense gratification, making money with no meaning, conquests of sex, and video games. It means you know how to breathe and how to be still in yourself during the course of a day—no matter what whirlwind is around you. Nothing is more masculine than being a deep force of consciousness in the face of life's ups and downs. This ability says to a woman or a more feminine-identified person that you can handle matters when the storm of energy and expression starts to rage and that you aren't going to change your direction because of the passing weather pattern.

And dating can be a place where you get to express that kind of consciousness in full. It's more *fun* that way. And part of enjoying dating and getting to feel a bigger sense of yourself as a man means having awareness, perspective, stability, and smart decision making. This all stems from your ability to breathe into your lower body, feel your legs, and find a center of gravity within yourself—preferably a couple of inches below the belly button, which will anchor you.

In the realm of modern dating, one thing men misunderstand is having sex with a woman and thinking she's not going to be attached. *Any* time you have sex with a woman and it's a somewhat enjoyable experience, that woman is going to become biochemically and energetically attached and connected to you . . . wait for it . . . forever. I know this may not seem true in the world of casual sex, but I'm telling you that it is. She may not know it herself, and—trust me—her feeling this way doesn't mean you have to marry her, but it's really, really important to know and understand that she feels this way. If you're having sex with men, this is different. It really only applies to woman-man sexual intercourse because a woman has certain parts of her energetic anatomy that are tuned for her receiving the information of your familial, lineal, and genetic codes in the case that you would become father to her child.

When you are kind, you like women, and want to respect them, or you simply just want to avoid drama, having sex with a woman you don't really want to have some kind of a relationship with, however casual, can create more harm than good. And it's important as an evolving man to have the wisdom to know which is when. Now, you can do *other* things on your one-night stand. But having penetrative sex with a woman is a 100 percent guaranteed way to trigger the attachment instinct in a woman or hurt her feelings because you as a man do not operate the same way biologically. We're trying to build a world of understanding between the sexes, and so more and more compassion for each other and the way we operate biochemically is necessary to bridge these gaps. And negotiating the dating scene in a deeper, more intelligent way does count and will make you stand out as a man of integrity.

In addition, having a deeper discernment and reverence around sexual engagement will accelerate the expansion of your consciousness. Yogi Bhajan gave this teaching around the power of sex to amplify or degenerate intelligence and awareness in a vast and cosmic sense.

> *Physical intercourse is called "The Bridge of Seven Constructions." You can elevate your physical, mental, and spiritual body seven times over if it is an intercourse of mind, body and soul—if it is sacred, if it is worthwhile. Otherwise, it is the dumbest thing to do.*
>
> —YOGI BHAJAN

Essentially, if you understand the power of sex, and enter into a sexual engagement with intelligence and respect and a bit of yogic science, you can up-level your consciousness sevenfold. However, if that space is not available to you, a random sex act, no matter how satisfying and passionate, can actually downgrade your awareness. If you're at all interested in merging your mind into the yogic heights of cosmic oneness, how you approach physical intimacy is an important place of focus.

If you're just out there to date, have fun. Remember, the whole point of dating is in many ways to become a better man who will attract higher-and-higher-quality partners. Becoming a pickup artist is a toxic mimic of what it means to be a true evolutionary man. So you might get some social praise for it, and you might get some satisfaction for your ego, but the bedrock of your integrity as a man does not feel fulfilled. Fulfillment comes from a relay of energy and experience between two or more people, and this relay, when done with some artistry, can be utterly powerful and inspiring for your purpose and direction on the planet. This is where relating with women will start to be healing and productive rather than habitually destructive, draining, and distracting.

A basic Yogi Bhajan teaching is that a woman has three forms, only one of which most men have been conditioned to relate to in our society—the physical form. But as many men know, no matter how hot her physical form is and how fun sex with her was in the moment, there's always a price to pay when you relate only to that singular part of her. Whether she gets angry that you've ditched her after sex, or she gets insecure and starts crazy texting you, or you realize shortly after sex that you're done with her and you feel subconsciously guilty or not good about yourself—it's ultimately not fulfilling.

In order to get true fulfillment from any interaction with a woman, you must relate to her spiritual and mental forms as well as her physical form.

Being a man is so much more satisfying and integrated than what you've

> *All three forms must support you.*
> *If one form of the woman supports*
> *you, it is no support at all.*
>
> —YOGI BHAJAN

been sold by the media, music culture, and society. Your essence is touched by the deeply fulfilling dance of both the direction of purpose and the emptiness of nothing that you've been hunting and craving your whole life. Even though by nature men are seeders, they are also simultaneously providers, lovers, counselors, rocks, and so much more. By acknowledging the forms of woman, you also are acknowledging all the facets of yourself and, in the process, beginning to embody these facets. The more you are a total expression, the more deeply initiated you become as a man. This integration, depth, and strength gives you instantaneously more attractiveness inside and out, no matter what your physical form.

If you're interested in a relationship, know this about yourself. Most men find relationships soothing in many ways, and some men even have a *craving* for commitment, as it brings them closer to themselves as focused, creative, living potential manifesters. Being in a committed relationship helps men experience strength, focus, and goodness. When you're dating with the intention of finding a partner, look for a woman who can really see you and support your purpose. There are a lot of beautiful women out there who are so shallow, they will ultimately waste your time and distract you from your path. Seek women who have the ability to reflect you and be a true inspiration, intuitive guide, and companion on your journey.

When you do meet someone like this, woo her by making her feel safe. She is looking for your *leadership*—physically, emotionally, and spiritually. She wants your decisiveness, direction, and true desire.

Leader is the most intelligent person. She doesn't care for your intellectual raps, she doesn't care for your ego flairs, she doesn't care for a lot of things. A leader is a very sacrificial, highly calculated, most sophisticated human behavior in relationship to a woman. And that is expected of every woman: to demand a man who can lead her, who can stimulate her.

—YOGI BHAJAN

She also is attracted to your integrity, which is just another way of saying your ability to find, make, and stick to your own attunement of truth! Your integrity shows when you are integrated and relaxed in the face of danger, change, or challenge. She'll be so attracted to you as a man when you are genuine, comfortable, and direct. Women always ultimately know when men are acting outside of their own integrity, and it's one of the biggest turnoffs. They will quickly begin to disrespect you and act subversively and passive-aggressively in response to this subtle misalignment.

MEN IN RELATIONSHIPS

As I wrote above, relationship is the greatest yoga. And commitment for a man is both a highly powerful spiritual exercise, one that will develop you as a true warrior, and a very difficult biochemical exercise because it is coded in your genetics to not particularly be monogamous. In many ways committed relationship goes against a hardwired part of a man's nature (the animal part), which is important for women to understand and have compassion for. There is a spectrum of realities in current relationship possibilities, meaning many people are experimenting with more-honest relationships that may or may not include monogamy. Relationships are changing more rapidly than ever before, and for both men and women, consciously discussing our limbic system programs, what brings us more joy, what works in the parameters of a particular relationship, are all worthwhile subjects to explore.

As the honesty, intimacy, and connection grow deeper, relationship starts to have the power to transform and bring both parties into a higher form of themselves. This is when the yoga, the practice, really gets juicy and rewarding. The opposite of that is when relationship brings out the worst in both partners, which can happen as well. Each person in a relationship is subconsciously trying to have a bigger experience of something, and usually it's not the best of each other. However you can *train* yourself to experience the best things about your lover and relationship then becomes fertile ground for your human and spiritual development as a man.

One thing to note is that a woman is always testing you. *Always.* Women, for better or for worse, need to make sure everything is safe. She doesn't believe that everything's fine because of her innately primal and active mind that is wired to see all the worst things that could happen in any scenario in order to protect the "home and children." So she is going to test you to make sure everything is secure. Be aware of these tests and keep steady. This requires some connection to your breath and also that which will never end. It's a deep spiritual practice to keep grounded when you are being tested by the ever-changing moon like feminine aspect of anyone's psyche—these feminine tests actually show up in all genders. It's just nature testing man—it's that primal.

If a woman doesn't fluctuate, she's male.
They fluctuate. Let them fluctuate.
A stable woman is very boring.

—YOGI BHAJAN

STROKE BREATH FOR STABILITY

POSTURE: Sit in easy pose. Bring the hands to heart level with the left palm facing down and the right palm facing up. The hands should be directly in front of the heart center, palms facing each other, with about four inches of space between the hands. It should be as though you are holding a softball in front of the heart.

EYES: Focus the eyes on the tip of the nose.

BREATH: Inhale through the nose in eight equal strokes. Exhale through the mouth in eight equal strokes. Make the breath pattern continuous—i.e., don't take breaks in between the inhale and exhale cycles. Use the mantra *Sa-Ta-Na-Ma* to measure the count.

TIME: 11 minutes

TO END: Inhale and hold the breath for thirty seconds. Exhale slowly through the nose. Relax.

Women naturally cycle their moods and their conscious psyches every two and a half days. In the media, this is characterized often as a woman's moodiness, but as a conscious man, you can relate to the cycles differently. It's not that she's moody—it's that her psyche is naturally in flux. So it's why one night she wants to just be mellow and watch movies, and then the next day she's a sex maniac, and then two days after that she wants to go to church, and then two days after that she's burning Bibles. I'm exaggerating here, but the point is, it's not menstrual, it's not hormonal, it's not something that can be regularized. It's just a woman's natural way. She is a powerful weather pattern that *changes*. And your challenge is to learn to be *steady*.

She's going to have a whole spectrum of experiences, thoughts, and emotions. Just be steady. She might get mad, throw a temper tantrum, or have a total meltdown. Just be steady. Yogi Bhajan said never to engage a woman in her negativity. So this kind of balance requires an unparalleled level of nervous system strength and mental neutrality. You can learn through some of the techniques in this book, especially anything that deepens your breath, to be able to stand strong, relaxed, and calm in the eye of the storm. However, Yogi Bhajan left the Stroke Breath for Stability on page 190 as a practice especially for men to create nerves of steel.

Now, this doesn't mean you don't get to have your own emotions or your own ups and downs. But it does mean that you don't fall into the trap of hers. She might be picking a fight. Just be steady. This is going to eventually calm her and return you both to relational bliss.

In addition, always trust a woman's intuition. Over the course of history, we've been programmed to think women are crazy or fragile minded and not worth listening to. Yogi Bhajan taught that bioenergetically women are sixteen times more [fill in the blank] than men—positive and negative. This means that women are sixteen times more neurotic, but it *also* means that women are sixteen times more data sensitive, sixteen times more intelligent about what to do with that data, and sixteen times more effective when taking action. So just *listen*. The smartest men in the world listen to a woman's intuition.

Whatever you do, do not add to a woman's insecurity, because it will make you miserable. An insecure woman is a terror to be with. She then will not be able to relate to your masculinity in a way that's enjoyable for you, and because you have enlarged her insecurity, she will make your life much less enjoyable to say the least. So don't undermine your woman. Do your best to support her and *praise* her.

> *In the joy of your life, if you really want to enjoy your living, you must get the spring of life, the nectar of life, from the projections of a woman.*
>
> —YOGI BHAJAN

If her projection is strong, self-loving, and stable, you will reap the benefit of this in your life. She will be able to support and nourish your purpose, and ultimately, this is one of the reasons you would be attracted to going deeper into a committed relationship with her. If she projects your greatness and holds that vision of you, her support and prayer is very powerful.

We're entering a new time when women are expected to be professional, hot, *and* feminine throughout the course of a day, not even mentioning motherhood or all the other roles that are required. They are running all manner of society—from companies to nation-states. Kicking butt and taking names. At the same time, they are moms, wives, cooks for their families, and neighborhood leaders. Sometimes men in relationship with these women can think, *Does she even need me?*

Every woman needs to feel feminine, to feel prized and loved. It doesn't matter if she's the next president of the United States or the best homemaker who ever lived. Above all, no matter how powerful your woman is, she wants to be cherished and protected. Do this for her, and so much treasure can grow between you. As a strong, independent woman myself, I can personally attest to the more outward, the more type A, the stronger your woman is—the more she *needs* your cherishing and allowing for her to relax into some experience of your inner stillness. She actually needs your depth, which requires some sort of meditative and contemplative practice to cultivate and maintain. These aspects of yourself are some of the most important things you can give her, and doing so *does* require practice, deeper breath, embodiment, and a clear mind. All of the practices I've given in this book will do this, but my favorite for men is Sat Kriya in the next chapter. Do it three to sixty-two minutes a day for clear, calm, grounded, purposeful action.

When Yogi Bhajan was asked how to inspire women spiritually, he said one word: "Action." Often, when men get into the comfort of relationship, women feel like men lose their edge of action, and start to slowly disrespect them for that. It's a slow poison, but over the years it will become the beginning of the end if you don't continue to sharpen your tools, your depth of self-inquiry, if you don't keep your heart open, your body healthy, and your spiritual connection alive. I'm not talking religion here—I'm talking whatever your personal god is—nature, exercise, creativity, sports, meditation. Whatever brings you closer to yourself and the cycle of life and death.

9. SEX Is Science

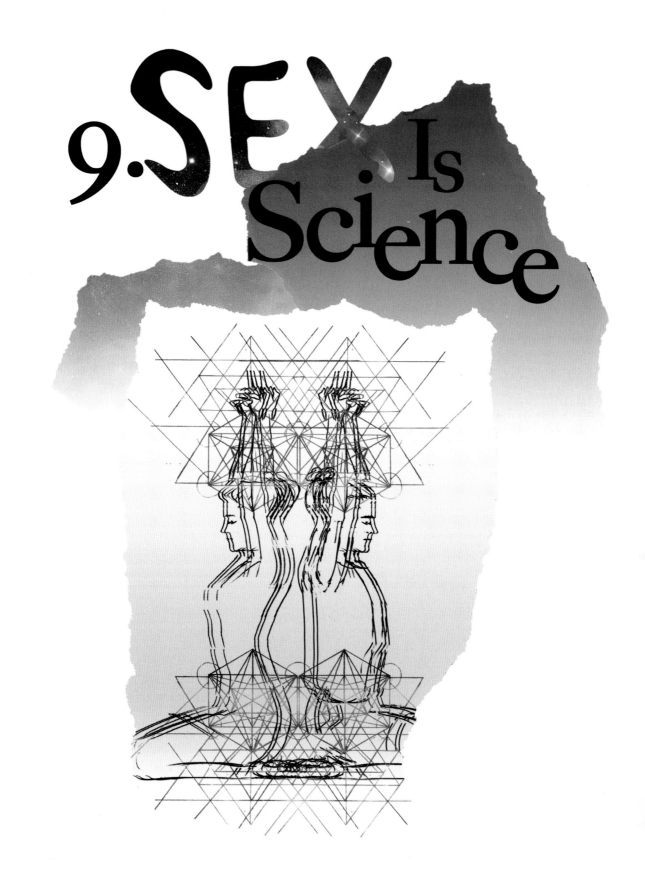

Sex is good. And it's a lifelong spiritual study if you choose to go deeper. Almost every human desires deeper sex as a metaphor for our infinite selves being expressed through the finite form and union with something greater and bigger.

Sex is healthy and important to a rich, developed, and embodied life. There are a lot of high spiritual teachings that create so much anxiety about sex that we have virtually no neutral, intelligent examples of what healthy, positive sex looks like, especially in the West. So let's just be clear: without advocating for going out and sleeping with everyone you know, sex is and can be godly. It creates humanity, and in its purest expression, sex is a gracious and spirit-filled act.

We live in a time when there is a massive polarity in our relationship to sexuality. The shame and fear-based, post-religious media leaves many women confused and locked down in the sexual pleasure centers. Yogi Bhajan, in his relentless effort to educate Westerners about what real sex is and does, said that USA stands for United Sex Allergy.

On the other side of the spectrum, what we are shown as "liberated sexuality" is another disguise for women's insecurity. These behaviors and beliefs are toxic mimics of what empowered sexuality actually looks like—women thrusting and sexualizing their *own* bodies, instead of being sexualized by society at large. Everywhere you look, men and women alike feel so empty—nothing is sacred, nothing holds any meaning, and it's just another ass or boob or whatever. This is a dead end, and many people end up in this empty space in their attempt to be healthy and sexually active humans. It's painful to use the power and potential of conscious sex and sensuality in a way that is ultimately harmful to yourself and others. *Making love* is kind of an outdated New Age term, but it does point to the whole *reason* we have sex—no matter if it's between friends with benefits or in a long-term committed relationship.

The reality is that sex *does* leave a lasting imprint on the body—especially women, and that can be negative *or* positive. What I would like to posit is that there is a possibility to discern how you're going to move through the sexual plane. We can be scientists and artists when it comes to our sexual experiences. We can be intelligent about our choices *and* know the techniques to take care of, be conscious of, and increase the enjoyment of both our own physioenergetic body and those we are sharing our body with. Depleting, negative, or dissatisfying sex *does* happen all the time, obviously, but it doesn't have to be that way. Instead, sex can be healthy and *exhilarating*!

INTELLIGENT SEX

The powerful, ancient teachings of Kundalini Yoga say again and again that we're householders and we're supposed to do household things. If we don't do household things, we get weird and out of sync. Sex is one of those household things!

Some of you have gone without sex for a prolonged period of time, which can be a powerful reset practice, but sex is ultimately a wonderful tool and science. As the human race recovering from the hangover of religious control mores on our society, we are fundamentally contracted and bound up around sex, and those knots of energy leak a lot of vitality from us physically, emotionally, and mentally. So healthy and frank conversations around sex are imperative to the whole culture—no matter how you identify your sexuality.

As I've touched on already, there are subtle and gross parts of our anatomy as whole beings, and one of the foundational pieces of the architecture of the human being is called an arcline. Yogic anatomy identifies two structures in the female aura called arclines. The first arcline runs from earlobe to earlobe, and it holds the magnetic patterns of your destiny, karma, and on the lowest common denominator, fate. Men also have this arcline. The *second* arcline, which occurs only in women, traces a radiant semicircle between the nipples. This one holds lineal information that you magnetically pass down to your offspring during the breast-feeding period. When you have sex with a man—even if it's just once—his whole aura and genetic lineal codes imprint onto that second arcline. Now, this information isn't to make you feel bad or ashamed if you had a couple of wild run-ins in whatever decade that was. But it is an important piece of information for men and women to understand when they are making intelligent decisions about sex.

My personal belief is that the reason we have this kind of imprinting mechanism is so that we can get the whole download of epigenetic, psychic, and lineal codes of the man. If, for instance, you *were* to have a baby with this man, you would have all of the lineal, genetic, and Akashic codings to pass down to the baby—vital information if you want to make a family. But that's a little inconvenient if you're having sex with someone you might not want to see ever again! In the past, these teachings were used in a very Victorian, lock-up-your-sex-drive way to scare women out of casual sex.

An intelligent and yogic way to create sexual empowerment, is that if you are *sensitizing* yourself in a certain way, there is a kind of *discernment* that will arise as you choose to maneuver through the sexual plane. You can enter into a sexual experience and make a decision for the experience to *not* imprint on your arcline very deeply. But this requires practice. At the same time, you can deactivate the imprints that are already there, but this too takes some work. So it's important to have the power of choice—so that we can make healthy decisions around how we deal with the imprints that are already there and how and when we take on new ones.

Part of why I'm interested in bringing awareness about the imprinting system is because those imprints take up valuable space in your arcline, crowding out the potential massive flow of additional prosperity and radiance. The arcline rules what you magnetize, or attract, into your life. The more radiant these spaces are, the better your chances to attract more radiant experiences, opportunities, people, and materials. And the clearer the arcline, the more the energy you have to live your highest destiny. Deactivating the imprints that you are carrying and creating more radiant circulation in this space is productive for a healthy and enjoyable life.

Luckily, we have a technology that deactivates those imprints.

YOGIC TECH FOR EMPOWERED SEX

One of my favorite arcline healing practices is the Cross-Hearted Kirtan Kriya meditation I gave in the previous chapter. This practice fortifies the auric structure and clears out anything imprinted there that you no longer wish to hold.

Another really powerful practice is Sat Kriya (given a little later in this chapter) or taking cold showers. I think we all know how taking a shower clears energy. There's an instinctive need to take a shower after visiting someplace gross or icky, even if you are not actually dirty. Or to shower after a breakup. But a cold shower washes away the energy more quickly and more

MEDITATION FOR THE ARCLINE AND TO CLEAR THE KARMAS

POSTURE: Sit in easy pose. Bend the arms at the elbows so that, in this starting position, the forearm is parallel to the ground and the upper arm is relaxed by the side. Palms are facing up, slightly cupped and floating above the knees.

EYES: Keep your eyes closed, gently focusing up and in at the brow point.

MANTRA AND MOVEMENT: *Wahe Guru, Wahe Guru, Wahe Guru, Wahe Jio.* Chant along with a recording of this mantra. In rhythm with the mantra, move the arms up and over the head as if you are scooping up water and tossing it over your shoulders. Keep the arms bent, and make sure the hands come up and over the ears when you bring them back behind you. In this way you clear both the breast arcline and the halo.

TIME: 11 to 31 minutes with practice

TO END: Inhale and stretch your arms back as far as possible. Hold for 15 seconds. Exhale and repeat twice more.

effectively *and* brightens the radiance of all ten bodies, which is something a regular hot shower just can't do as well.

I also really love the Meditation for the Arcline and to Clear the Karmas given on the previous page. It takes a bit more time and some fortitude, but it's *totally* worth it.

PLEASURE AND EXHILARATION

If you decide that you want to have sex, whether that's with your partner of twenty years or with someone you are spending some shorter amount of time with, you deserve to have fun and be in your body and enjoy your vitality!

Having a system that is ready and able to receive pleasure is just as important as making choices about who you decide to ride off into the sunset with. There are a lot of strange representations and models of sexuality in the media that don't necessarily lead to real pleasure. I say this because more than 60 percent of women report sexual dissatisfaction. So if these media representations had *any* veracity, wouldn't we be having *more* orgasms instead of the seemingly normal trend of faking them? This type of dissatisfaction leads to deep resentment and anger in women, and eventually to the breakdown of a healthy relationship. The divorce rate interestingly is now hitting about the same percentage! *This is not a coincidence.*

At the same time, the multibillion-dollar pharmaceutical industry is banking on you and your partner or partners losing sexual vitality at a certain age—like your sex drive just stops, or your vagina dries up, or he can't get it up anymore. Sexual dysfunction and low vitality are products of modern living and misuse of our sexuality. Yogis know you can have sexual vitality into your hundreds!

The benefits of a healthy, satisfying sex life are *many,* and I want them for you! So let me share with you the yogic wisdom for exciting, intoxicating, invigorating, and responsible sex!

FOUNDATIONAL SEXUAL KNOW-HOW

For really good, satisfying, fortifying sex, there are two important things to keep in mind:

1. For really delicious sex, avoid doing it between 3:00 A.M. and 6:00 A.M. Because of the position of the sun with the Earth during these hours, it is a very sensitive time of day, and sex at this time can be very psychologically and physically depleting. It's a good time to meditate but not a good time to *do it*.

2. If you want to have a maximum sexual experience, avoid sex within three hours after eating. A full stomach numbs your system, setting the stage for a subpar sexual experience. Engaging in sex on a semi-empty stomach allows the amount of pleasure you experience to amplify tenfold!

STRESS AND SEX

If you find that sex is stressful for you, there are a lot of yogic techniques to release your anxiety and open up the depth of your sexual enjoyment. One of these is to have an awareness of the seventy-two-hour buildup that happens before you actually engage in the act. It may seem a bit over the top to start the energetic foreplay for sex three days ahead of time, but biochemically, emotionally, and energetically, that's how far in advance sex starts. And if you are aware of it, you can start mentally and physically relaxing during that three-day window and doing practices that allow you to be more present and in your body, which will improve and deepen your experience in powerful and more erotic ways. Trust me, three days of foreplay can get *really hot*. During this window, practice deep breathing, exercise, eat well, flirt with your partner, and wear clothes that make you feel good.

FIFTEEN-MINUTE SEX MEDITATION

NOTE: This is really about moving the energy and smoothing the blocks that have gotten all twisted up in you, so that you can enjoy a healthy, balanced, clean sex drive and deep pleasure and energy during the act.

POSTURE: Sit and place the soles of your feet together in butterfly pose. Bring your hands in front of your body.

EYES: Keep your eyes closed, gently focusing up and in at the brow point.

BREATH: Let the breath self-regulate, and bounce your body up and down while thinking about sex.

MENTAL FOCUS: Whatever comes forward here, please don't repress it. Just let it come up. Clear out the kinks and the stagnancy and the twists. Consciously get horny and breathe. Heal yourself. Feel joyful about your vitality and your body and its ability to experience sexual pleasure.

TIME: 15 minutes

TO END: Inhale, exhale, breathe, and let the energy circulate. Relax.

Every relationship benefits from this awareness. You can start sexting back and forth with a new "friend" seventy-two hours before your next date to build up to something really enjoyable when you next see each other. For a man, sex begins in the pituitary gland—you may be surprised, his third eye. This gland is what commands the actual physical sexual act. If you can communicate with a man through his third eye, you'll get much further, and the written word goes right into the third eye.

If you're in a long-term relationship, this seventy-two-hour warm-up period is a beautiful practice to keep alive. It makes sex deeper while keeping things exciting. It's especially good awareness if you're an older couple and your man has lost some libido. This three-day pre-sexual window will help your man's pituitary gland and wake him up a little bit. Then you can enjoy something powerful and electric, like you did when you first met! It is possible to re-create the biochemistry that was naturally secreting between you two in the early days of your relationship.

CLASSICAL SAT KRIYA

POSTURE: Sit in rock pose with your buttocks on the heels. Bring the arms overhead, stretching from the armpits, and then steeple the index fingers, and interlace the other fingers. Women cross the left thumb over the right; men do the opposite.

EYES: Keep your eyes closed, gently focusing up and in at the brow point.

BREATH AND MANTRA: Breathe naturally and chant the mantra *Sat Nam* out loud. On *Sat*, pull your rectum, sex organs, and navel point up and in. On *Nam* release the lock. Continue.

TIME: 3 to 11 minutes

TO END: Inhale, stretch more, and pull your rectum, sex organs, and navel point up and in. Exhale and release. Repeat. Then inhale, exhale, hold the breath out, and stretch more. Inhale and relax the arms and gently lower yourself onto your back. Ideally relax on the back for the same amount of time that you practiced Sat Kriya. Or at least for a couple of minutes if you don't have a lot of time.

If you feel really sexually locked down, it's a beautiful gift to yourself and your world to start clearing blockages so that you can conduct a greater amount of pleasure and energy through your body. Maybe there was a lot of sexual repression in your family, or perhaps you had some deeply negative experiences around sex earlier in your life. Some trauma or closure is blocking your ability to enjoy sex and your ability to connect with another person. One such yogic technique for healing sexual repression and dysfunction is the Fifteen-Minute Sex Meditation (page 202).

By far, the best yogic technique for healing sexual dysfunction and opening up the flow of pleasure in your body is a practice called Sat Kriya. This will clear out any of the psychic and emotional baggage in your pleasure centers, release the flow of energy in this area, and consciously connect the lower energy centers with the higher ones. It's a total systemic upgrade practice.

SAT KRIYA: BATHTUB VARIATION

There are many variations of Sat Kriya. This one is really warming and opening for the whole body, including your sexual organs.

DIRECTIONS: Fill a tub with warm water. Sit on your heels and do Sat Kriya as given above for up to 15 minutes. Then lie down in the tub and relax.

Do this regularly to release tension and sexual frozenness, or just to get your energy moving.

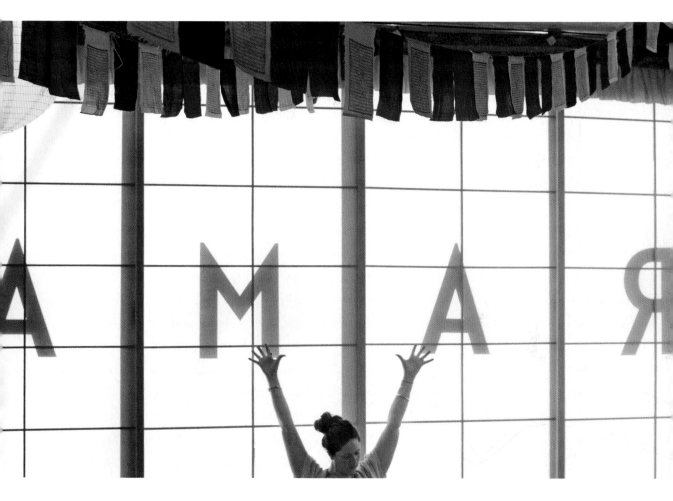

MAXIMUM ORGASM PRACTICES

My all-time favorite technology for healing sexuality and opening up deep pleasure for a woman is the *mulbhand*. In the medieval courts in China, the geishas, dakinis, and tantrikas used body-lock practices as part of intimate maintenance. Performing muscular isolations with their pelvic muscles allowed them to stay sexually vital *and* sexually healthy into old age. Women in the courts of China were so strong in their pelvic floor muscles that they could lift the weights just by contracting their vaginal walls, just as if they were competing in a sport! When you start to isolate and strengthen the pelvic floor, you change the level of pleasure you can experience in sex.

When you lose pelvic floor strength, however—say, after having surgery or after giving birth—a lot of other physical and psychoemotional things happen. A strong pelvic floor allows you to feel empowered; it is fortifying. A strong pelvic floor will allow you to feel more comfortable and engaged in your sexuality. A strong pelvic floor also physiologically allows your body to experience more satisfying, more exalted orgasms.

Many women are unaware of the fact that there are different levels and kinds of orgasms. The deepest kind of orgasm is called cervical and besides its being full-body sublime, it can happen without having sex, just from engaging in beauty, art, or nature. Like smelling a flower or seeing a beautiful sunset. In fact a lot of women report having cervical orgasms outside of intercourse. And that's how *sensitive* it is possible to become. When you are that sensitive, when you get into an actual sexual situation, every *touch* is orgasmic. There will be much less sexual dissatisfaction. Your whole body and subtle body system will pulsate with waves of pleasure and eroticism. Powerful.

Most people are only having "bucket sex," as Yogi Bhajan called it. Like there's a bucket and a stick. You're just stirring around. There's no science behind it. The word *Tantra* actually has nothing to do with sex—one level of Tantra is about a subtle body union that *can* happen in sex (mostly it doesn't happen the way sex is often practiced), but it can also happen everywhere else too. The point is that if you use the subtle yogic techniques of connecting deeper to the whole experience of finite connecting to infinite—Tantric teachings of union and subtly—and apply them to sex, it will be a lot more satisfying. And those subtle body experiences can be opened up with these practices.

The *mulbhand* is very effective for opening up this kind of subtlety and sensitivity. It seems like an all-too-simple, and maybe too esoteric practice, but if you practice this body lock daily for even just a week it's astounding the level of vitality, body confidence, and pleasure in all things that gets released. The *mulbhand* also serves as a powerful healing tool for women who have had issues with their periods, painful sex, urinary tract infections, dilation and curettage, abortions, fibroids, cervical scar tissue from having children, sexual traumas, or any other chronic issues.

Sat Kriya is the most powerful practice that uses the *mulbhand* for pelvic toning and, if you don't want to practice it every day, it's an impressively useful part of your seventy-two-hour pre-sex warm-up to get things flowing. This practice *will* increase the depth and satisfaction of the sexual experience. It is also really great for postmenopausal women who are in or are looking for romantic relationships. The *mulbhand* will help maintain pelvic strength, which will allow you to remain sexually vital *and* sexually healthy.

Sex is meant to provide you with energy, vitality, joy, and wellness. Let these practices open up more positivity in your sex life and a renewed, sustained sense of pleasure in every facet of your life.

IO.
PROSPERITY

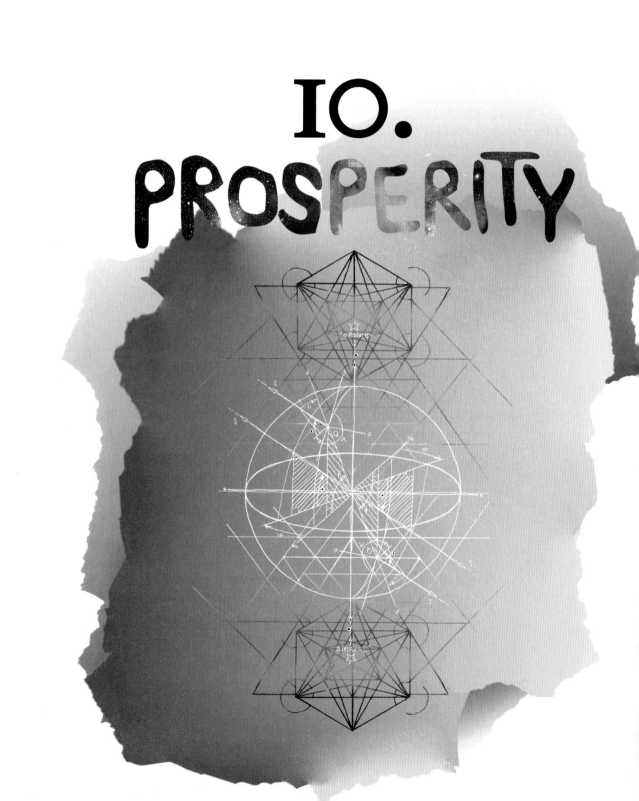

One of the things that astounds me about Kundalini Yoga is the wealth of prosperity practices that not only change your abundance on many levels but also your perception of resources. Kundalini Yoga and Meditation enhances your ability to handle success by strengthening the nervous system and to enjoy the richness of all aspects of living a full and experienced life. Practicing helps you be grounded as you become more materially and spiritually abundant—the gains and losses. It gives you what Yogi Bhajan called "dealing power"—the ability to deal with whatever is in front of you with finesse, resourcefulness, and enjoyment.

A lot of people have financial success and are miserable. Some people have a lot of freedom and creativity but have nothing to show for it, and the stress of financial issues weighs them down. But there doesn't have to be a chasm between personal fulfillment and personal finances, unencumbered creativity and unimaginable success. You are allowed to have financial wellness, freedom, and spontaneity, all while growing into your knowing of yourself and your creativity.

I think part of the confusion is that we in the West have been promised fulfillment exclusively in the form of money. And I can tell you that you won't find your deepest fulfillment through money alone. It can *help* you help yourself and others, but we have lots of examples of people who have *lots* of material abundance and *no fulfillment* whatsoever. However, just because the truest fulfillment doesn't come through money doesn't mean you shouldn't have any money at all *or* that you shouldn't enjoy the abundance of money, love, health, and creativity, among many of life's other pleasures.

Kundalini Yoga has multiple techniques for actualizing and bringing true, tangible wealth into reality. But before we get into how real wealth is created and how money can be utilized and contained, I think it's important to talk about the bigger picture, specifically how your whole relationship with money is organized around the inflow and outflow in your life—your prosperity.

PROSPERITY

In reality, it doesn't matter how much money you have. All that matters is your *relationship* to your own abundance. And this relationship is a *thought form*. You could be a total billionaire, with bank accounts in the Caymans and the latest Lamborghini and all the trappings of a wealthy person, and *still* relate to your wealth from the point of view of scarcity. Many people do. They have all the money in the world, and they still feel poor. They still feel like, *Any minute it could all be taken away*, or *It's still not enough*, or *Someone else has more than I do*. And this is from someone who, by all external realities, is *not* poor. But they live in *a poverty experience*.

Whatever scarcity you've been relating to—it's an absolute untruth. There is a real fear-mongering situation in our mass-consumption society that wants you to believe that there is not enough. Images of starvation, images of lack and decay. You start to believe, *There's not enough, there's not enough, there's not enough.*

That's a false broadcast that there's not enough. It's not true. A third of our food supply is thrown away every year. At *least*. There are not citable *reasons* why this happens, but it seems to me to be part of an agenda to create more fear and lack on the planet. There are all sorts of weird excuses that are given as legitimate—but there are many holes in those arguments. There are many reasons, however, to keep the population feeling and believing that there is not enough, and those thoughts create vibrational reality.

"They" say there isn't enough, but there *is* enough if we are smart, resourceful, and collaborative.

Poverty consciousness can be so deep and can rule every single action of every day. It may not show up in the classical ways—fear-based concerns about money—it may show up in *other* ways. For instance, you might have an impoverished way of relating to yourself and to the world. You might feel like you have no time (time poverty), you might fear taking risks (safety poverty), or you could be stingy in your love for others or your love for yourself (love poverty). However it shows up, this poverty consciousness is draining your energy in a way that you are not able to deliver to the planet what you came to deliver. Then you can't experience the fulfillment of delivering your unique creative payload. And if you don't have fulfillment, it won't matter how many millions of dollars you have or don't have.

Take a look at all the ways in which you engage in your world in an impoverished manner, and make a mental or physical list. The mind has to be trained to organize your thoughts in a certain way if you want to inherit the respective treasures, whatever that may mean to you in this lifetime. There are yogic prerequisites to the enjoyment of these treasures, though: you need to be strong enough and generous enough, and you have to *widen* your capacity, perspective, nervous system, and radiance to lay claim to the wealth of human experience there is to be had and enjoyed.

Widening is a combination of actual biophysiological nervous system strength *and* an emotional and psychological perspective. So it's a little like stretching your physical body. You are stretching your nervous system in order to receive the literally immense wave of prosperity that's coming at you. If your nervous system is only able to conduct a limited amount of pleasure, happiness, joy, and prosperity, then no matter how much of these things are available to you, you can only experience as much of them as your nervous system can uptake.

And you have to widen your perspective. If you have the nervous system to conduct more prosperity but your psychology and your emotional habits are still scarcity oriented, then you won't tap into the full capacity of the nervous system, which limits your experience of, and appreciation for,

PRANIC ENERGY MULTIPLIER

POSTURE: Sit in easy pose. Rest your hands in your lap with your fingers interlaced.

EYES: Keep your eyes open. In this meditation, this is a direct requirement. Do not close the eyes.

BREATH: Breathe in through pursed lips as though you were sipping from a straw. Rhythmically sip air through your mouth in strokes, about one per second. Just keep taking in air continuously without thinking about the exhale. Just keep inhaling, inhaling, and inhaling. Take in more, more, and even more. More than you think you can. The exhale will be automatic. Just take in more. You're trying to inhale for the full length of the meditation, which is five minutes.

TIME: 5 minutes

TO END: Inhale, hold the breath for as long as possible. Exhale and relax.

abundance. It's like having a computer but not turning it on. You'll never access the Internet.

One way we widen our perspectives is by starting to look at life as a whole spectrum, life as a whole journey—life as a whole blessed, blessed, blessed, blessed incarnation. It's just so big and vast and beautiful and such a precious gift. When we begin to relate with the immensity of our entire being, we can move methodically, step by step, in the direction of our greatest fulfillment. When we *widen*, we experience less tension. When we experience less tension, we can begin to relax deeper and deeper, and then more things can *happen* for us.

There's a really great Kundalini exercise called the Pranic Energy Multiplier that creates a strength and a widening in the nervous system that literally increases your ability to hold more. Most people who are stuck in a poverty experience are naturally calibrated to that energetic space and are afraid to hold more. This meditation forces you to get stronger and more capable of conducting the in- and outflow of energy.

COLD, HARD CASH

I believe it's powerful to create *money*. Money is just energy and can be a sign that there's good flow happening in your life. Sometimes the New Age prosperity conversations can get a little etheric, so I think it's important to also get hard-core, 3-D, practical indications of your prosperity.

I grew up in the thick of the 1980s New Age movement with some beautifully spiritual people. These were people who understood the fundamentals of reality, were interested in building a new society, had the consciousness to do it, but couldn't get their finances in order. Year after year it was the same thing. They didn't have any money. It's just another guru, another healing art modality, another message from the interstellar realm, but no prosperity.

It's now thirty years later, and they are still trying to get their Reiki business off the ground, which is disappointing, because if you want to build something, you need some material wealth to do it. And in order to *really* help yourself and others, you have to be stable: emotionally, physically, mentally, and *materially*.

The good news is, if we can get conscious about money, if we can spelunk the terrain of subconscious booby traps around money and *disengage* some of this stuff, this is a real and practical area where we can make major spiritual and material progress. Yogi Bhajan called money one the heaviest thing on the planet earth.

But ultimately, money is just energy. All Kundalini Yoga practices take you spelunking in the depths of your neurology, where the blackouts are—where we go unconscious. We reprogram the weirdness we often picked up from our parents and grandparents around money and prosperity, the shame, fear, guilt. When we take the time to do this, it can actually change this primal relationship with feeling enough and that we have enough and all the ways that shows up in our lives. When balanced and strengthened, this enoughness can make us much more solid, grounded people on all levels.

MANIFESTING MONEY

Kundalini Yoga is an effective means to change your whole inflow and outflow experience. This yoga is a *command* technology that allows you to send vibrational messages to the biofeedback system of the Universe, with all the spectrum of potential realities, that you are *ready* for more. This is a *command* that you are ready for a nicer place to live, a better job, a healthy relationship, massive amounts of cash . . . whatever. There is no lack of supply, there's lack of *demand*.

When I opened the first RA MA Institute in Venice Beach, California, I spent many early morning meditations not in some New Age bliss, but getting real and commanding that this studio be successful. *I showed up. I built the studio. Now bring the success! Make this happen!* My destiny had called me to build this studio, and many of us know that the brick-and-mortar business in America is not an easy prospect, especially in urban areas like Los Angeles. Something bigger than just me built these studios, and I took major professional, personal, and financial risks to do so—and so I really demanded in my practice and meditations that those higher forces also provide the means for them to stay open and thrive!

So, I've made it a daily practice to live by Yogi Bhajan's teaching that there is no lack of supply; there is *lack of demand and lack of command.* This is how it works: you use the energy cultivated in the yogic practices to command what it is you want. Then, once you've commanded what you want, open up a space to create it and manifest it. And *then* . . . you have to be able to handle it! The amount of material or spiritual wealth that you can hold is directly related to how much your nervous system can handle.

And this is really where the problem is. We can get what we want—we all know that. We've all read, or seen or at least heard about, *The Secret.* We know manifestation is possible. But when people manifest, the real call to action and destiny happen. How we behave, then, in the trenches of actually getting what we want is a very interesting and powerful thing.

I want you to be successful and then be *happy* about being successful. A lot of people are successful and then they're *not* happy about it. Isn't that funny? There are a lot of miserable successful people. Part of this is because when a person moves up into a certain kind of success, we trigger all sorts of self-sabotage programs. Some of these failure switches come from the way we were raised or the way we were educated. There's a kind of peer consciousness that gets programmed in the family and in the school system that if you succeed in a certain way or show up in a certain way, you're showing off. You don't want to one-up your classmates or your friends or your siblings. Or in some cases it's the exact opposite programming—that you're always trying to compete and one-up, and this creates an anxiety and numbness that can turn into drug and alcohol use or other self-sabotages as an adult. And while we want to have healthy relationships in all those areas, none of them should be an inhibiting factor on your success. Yet all of this starts to creep up once you've reached certain goals or achievements in your life.

Even more and deeply so, a lot of failure mechanisms were programmed in utero. When our mothers were pregnant, many of them were stressed or feeling some kind of abandonment from their husbands or, for those conceived in the 1960s, on some kind of amphetamine . . . the list goes on and on. Any kind of stresses we may have experienced in utero go into our neurological programming and create short-circuits in the nervous system and blackouts that are triggered throughout our lives, particularly when we reach for something higher.

We are progressing and progressing, and all of a sudden we've hit a subconscious glass ceiling. The self-sabotage program has been activated. Sometimes this has to do with a fear of how successful we can be without threatening those who gave us life—like our mothers or fathers. Some parents, and this is really true, were frightened in a very primal way of the intelligence and power of the soul that they were giving life to. It's a natural progression to be far more advanced than those who gave us life. This is evolution at work. And they could tell subconsciously when we were in the womb that we were more advanced than them, which triggered *their* failure and success patterns. As a result, they became nervous that we would show them how backward they were, nervous that they couldn't actually take care of souls like ours. So they programmed us very subconsciously.

Those programs are so innate and heavy and hard to see that most people live their whole lives without recognizing they are in patterns that aren't even their own. Those patterns are from society, the collective consciousness, and the preprogramming of our parents.

So it's not a question of whether you're going to hit this success barrier; it's a question of when. Make no mistake: you *will* hit it. But that doesn't mean you can't break through these blocks. Look at hitting them as good news. It's good news when you hit some kind of bump in your subconscious around your success because that means things are happening. Then how do we deal with it? We have so many examples of very successful people with a lot of notoriety who have not taken care of their nervous system and therefore aren't handling their success and their fame very well.

Many celebrities in our culture are a great example of this. These are people who have hugely structured radiant bodies that have the ability hold massive prosperity, talent, beauty, and success. However, their nervous systems aren't strong, and the wattage of the fame and prosperity literally fries them. That's why you see celebrities in a downward spiral all over the media.

Unfortunately, there are countless examples of what it looks like to *command* and *receive* and then not be able to handle the prosperity in a long-term graceful and healthy way. We have very few role models who handle success well. And part of why I feel these prosperity teachings and practices are so important is so we can become individuals who have success and can *handle it*—with dignity, generosity, intelligence, and empowerment.

Once we command the prosperity into reality, we then have to have the *nervous system* and the *grit* to be able to contain it. Major prosperity is a big wave of energy. Even though it's positive, you still need to be strong enough to ride the wave.

Nothing short-circuits your nervous system like anger and impatience, so when it comes to receiving and handling prosperity gracefully, a really powerful practice is this Fists of Anger exercise. Fists of Anger detoxes the pent-up energy of frustration and self-hatred that's inside most people on the planet. That anger actually prevents all the blessings from coming to you, so you need to release it for the prosperity to have more flow. This breath also releases such a current of radiance that the nerves start to be able to conduct more wattage. Your capacity widens, your energy clears, and your grit develops.

FISTS OF ANGER

POSTURE: Sit in easy pose or rock pose. Make your hands into fists with your thumb on the inside, touching the mound of flesh below your pinky.

EYES: Keep your eyes closed, gently focusing up and in at the brow point.

BREATH: Do a powerful Breath of Fire through an O-shaped mouth. Take one arm overhead like a backstroke and then the other, alternating and using your frustration to fuel the movement.

TIME: 3 minutes

TO END: Inhale, hold the breath, interlace your fingers, and stretch your arms up with your palms facing the ceiling. Imagine yourself surrounded with white shimmering light. Exhale but keep your arms stretched up. Repeat twice more inhaling, holding the breath as you stretch and feel yourself surrounded with white shimmering light, white upon white. Exhale and relax.

AURIC ROOTING

Wealth, actual material prosperity, takes groundedness. What I mean by groundedness doesn't have anything to do with a hustle mentality or even not dreaming big. What I mean by groundedness is also known in yoga as *auric rooting*.

The idea of *auric rooting* can feel a little foreign to some people. For others, you're going to intuitively get the sense right away of what this means.

Here's how it works: When you get sensitive to your more subtle bodies, which will come in time, you can start to command the more subtle energetic parts of you. Auric rooting occurs when you send your focus into the earth beneath you, literally commanding the energy body through the heel of each foot physically. The amount of material wealth that you can hold is directly related to how deeply your aura can take root.

Auric rooting gives you the ability to be sensitive in a way to physically embody a higher caliber of energy, which *is* prosperity. We know that you can be prosperous in experience and that this has nothing to do with money. However, if you want *actual* money, then you also need to be able to recognize the opportunities that are going to make these actual resources available to you. That recognition and groundedness is essential to the more dense aspects of 3-D prosperity.

Because money is an element of the earthern plane, the deeper your auric field goes into the Earth, the more sensitive you will be to *opportunities* that present themselves to you and the right action around those opportunities. Then you can act on the opportunity, and actual, tangible abundance is a good indication you are going in the right direction. Forget aura photography (a love of mine) and analyzing what colors show up. This is how the somewhat esoteric becomes practical and tangible.

GENEROSITY AND PROSPERITY

Ultimately, one of the foundational pieces around business, success, money, and profit is delivering from a space of *true giving*. There's power when you come from a space of compassion and care. When serving humanity comes before the bottom line, there is a wave of gratitude from the collective consciousness, and that's more *powerful* and profound than you can imagine. It is therefore more *profitable*. There are now countless examples of *thriving* companies that built themselves on profit sharing, corporate wellness, and philanthropy. The wellness industry and its increasing market share is in one way an example that business based on health and happiness in some way is the new economic model.

FULFILLMENT

Inextricably woven into matters of money and prosperity is the bigger, more expansive, more life-affirming arena of fulfillment. Something *deep* in us is looking for true fulfillment. It's one thing to have success. We live in a country where there's *lots* of success and very little fulfillment. *Very little.* There is a big chasm between success and fulfillment.

Most of you reading this book are not interested in success for success's sake. You're motivated by something bigger, like powerful experiences and serving humanity. That's why there's an emptiness when you just go after success. You are sensory. You want to enjoy abundance, but you're not here for the hustle.

I think it's very important that we start to understand that fulfillment is different than success. Success is an external experience, whatever your version or conditioned version of that looks like. From a very early age, we have all kinds of programs conditioned in us about what success looks like or what it doesn't look like. You get into the rat race, and you get the degree, and the job, and the promotion, and the raise, and the house, and the car, and the thing, and the other things, and all the other things.

Even if it's "success"—even if it's in the model of success, even if there's monetary success—it's not a fulfillment of the soul. It's not a fulfillment of destiny. We all want true human fulfillment, not just some idea of success, and that's a whole other level. Humans don't feel fulfilled unless they feel like they are delivering what they are meant to deliver or create during their lifetime.

And your busy-ness, anxiety, depression, neurosis, and narcissism are certainly not going to fulfill you.

We are inherently wired for happiness. We're not wired to be depressed. Everything in our system is wired to be happy—and not only happy but also fulfilled, which creates true happiness.

AXIS AND ORBIT

In the householder traditions of Kundalini Yoga, Yogi Bhajan referred to the axis and the orbit as the biofeedback mechanisms of your internal spiritual spring and external material abundance. True fulfillment is when the axis and the orbit work together so that we actually feel like we are delivering what we are meant to deliver—it's intrinsically connected to our creativity as creative beings.

Your success can really take any shape, any container. It doesn't really matter what it looks like. It matters what your experience is. What does *experience* mean? Feeling a sense of achievement, purpose, and happiness. And most people will find that they are experiencing a level of satisfaction that they call success when two yogic aspects are in place and balanced: the *axis* and the *orbit*.

Axis is your internal alignment. How you organize your identity, priorities, and your mission. It's your inner conviction. Yogi Bhajan's teaching on the axis is this: when your mind and being are centered on the right axis, you *will* be happy whether you are rich or poor. *Orbit* is your outward sphere of influence. It's what you do in the world—how you choose to circulate in the material arena and how you choose to serve others. Yogi Bhajan says when your being is circulating in your right orbit, you will be rich whether or not you are happy.

To have success, fulfillment, and prosperity, you want to be on both your right axis and your right orbit. Because when both are strong and in harmony, you will be abundant, prosperous, and happy!

The best way to start to get a sense of your personal orbit and axis is to gain a deeper sensory relationship with inner and outer spheres of experience. Just go deeper within during your meditations or connect deeper with your breath. *And* simultaneously project farther *out*. From the deeply rooted space within, project out into the Cosmos—project into the far reaches of the Universe. Keep pressing at the bounds of your awareness and the ability of your psyche and whole being to participate on a grander scale and scheme.

When you train yourself in this way—to expand and contract simultaneously, just as everything in nature does—you begin to align with the natural order of things. Right action, creativity, and your response to the inflow and outflow of your life become much more artful and in sync. This flow is the baseline of your perceiving your life in a more harmonious and prosperous way and enjoying the depth and velocity of your soul's deeper yearning for varied experience in this lifetime—which ultimately is the call that must be answered for true prosperity.

Prosperity Tratakum

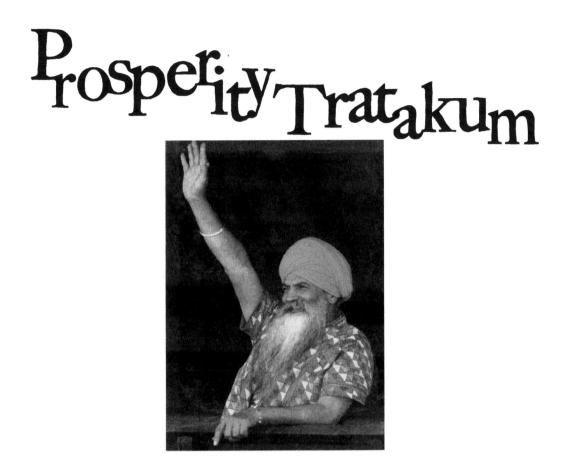

"And this is another moment where I might have raised my hand by mistake. So they took it on a picture and on the reverse side they printed the calendar of the 1998 events. This small picture is not the picture of a man. It is the picture of the Mahan Tantric. Now let me define it. The crossroads of energy of the psyche balances out at the heart center of the Mahan Tantric. So, it is a picture on paper, but sometimes it works wonders. If you cannot do anything for yourself, keep it in your purse. You'll be shocked. And if you get a lot of money and a lot of happiness, share it. Don't be selfish and alone, that's not fair, is it? So, somebody knew the facts and the scientific truth about it. You see this is how the universe is. Carry it with you. When you take it out, look at it, mentally project the word 'Victory' from your third eye and you shall surely prosper."

—YOGI BHAJAN

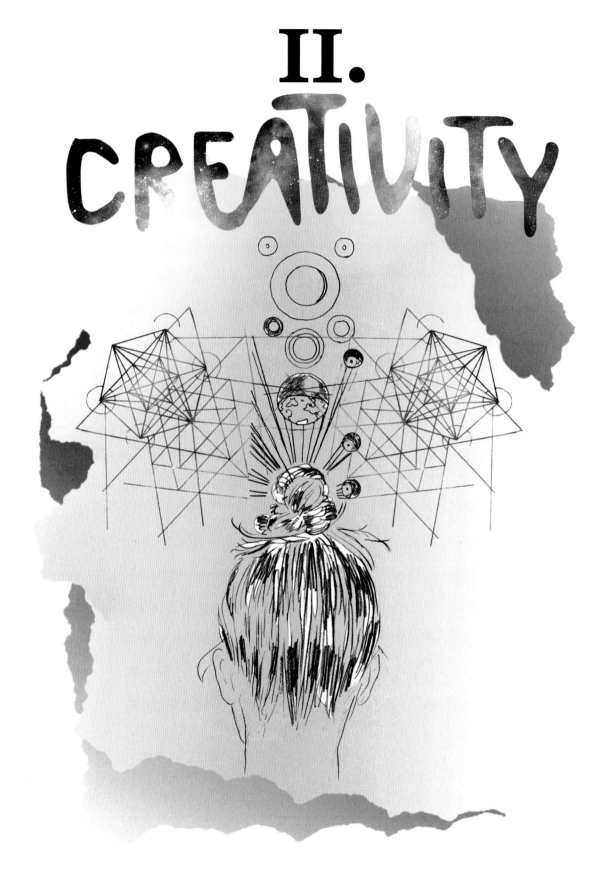

II.
CREATIVITY

I believe and constantly teach that creativity is the antidote to the mental bankruptcy and emotional emptiness of the Technology Age. If you create something and you are creative every single day, you're not going to feel the same level of emptiness that is crippling so many humans in modern life. We are born to create, so when we create we are happy and then we treat each other better. That in and of itself is revolutionary.

The whole Universe is awaiting you to step into your creative destiny. That doesn't have to look like traditional art. It can only really look like *your* creative destiny. And whether you think of yourself as an artist or you think of yourself as a businessperson or a parent . . . all of these are creative acts.

The very act of living is a creative act. Yogi Bhajan talked about crafting your life as a work of art. He said that you should walk in your life with such radiance that people say, "Wow! What a wonderful thing," the same way they exclaim about art in a gallery. You are both the product of creation and its creator. And creating the things that you know you need to create in this life—and a little bit of yoga and meditation—will give you the energy to have a truly happy life. And we truly *need* happy people on the planet. There are so many who are unfulfilled and unhappy that we have to balance the scales.

Part of the profundity of these practices is that they activate and facilitate the creative power in you, and this is an incredibly important part of you having the tools to live invincibly. The world is dying under the stagnancy and fear of doing anything new or taking risks—literally dying from the prosaic solutions for environmental rehabilitation to the total cowardice around restructuring the political economy. If we don't inject some new artistry soon, we won't be enjoying this Earth for much longer. And if we take the same amount of creativity and invention that's being used to destroy ourselves and the planet to instead create what Chögyam Trungpa Rinpoche called "enlightened society"—one based on the values of creativity, compassion, and community—then it is possible to get ourselves out of this mess we have created. But not without some true human ingenuity and creative genius.

Inseparable from the demand for activated creativity is the urgency for a new method of inspiration. A lot of times when we think of creativity, we

> *It is now highly feasible to take care of everybody on Earth at a "higher standard of living than any have ever known." It no longer has to be you or me. Selfishness is unnecessary. . . . War is obsolete. . . . It is a matter of converting the high technology from weaponry to livingry.*
>
> —R. BUCKMINSTER FULLER

frame it only as a product of angst or suffering, or from certain negative polarities that we experience on the planet. So much of art, and really any form of creativity if you think about, is some kind of masturbatory emanation of that artist's pain and suffering. This does *nothing* for a world so badly in need of imagination and new vision. That creative act born out of negative friction is just a compulsive habit, which *limits* real creativity.

Time to rework our concepts of what it means to be a creator on the planet and embody artistic clarity and creativity; the world needs your particular intelligence and unique perspective in whatever arena you can offer it. As a parent, an accountant, or a musician—your creativity is needed. We can learn to channel these natural impulses in a healing and progressive way so that whatever realm our creativity impacts, it's a fulfillment and a gift to the world rather than a singular manifestation of pain and continuation of our prolific neuroses.

DHARMA ART

At our core, our soul and our intelligence are inherently creative. As a businessperson, a yogi, and a teacher, I approach all of my tasks in a day to create works of art.

How do art and spirituality relate? I feel that the closest you can ever actually get to devotion, worship, God, and spiritual experience is through the pure creative act. The rest of the pomp and circumstance is ultimately just spiritual materialism. The real spirit shows up in the experience of creation. However, so many of us are afraid of our creativity, or at some point or another, we've been told that it's not valid or worthy.

Popularized by one of my favorite spiritual masters, Chögyam Trungpa Rinpoche, dharma art is essentially art that is in alignment with your spiritual development and a *nutritive* addition to the world. It's art as an outpouring of your spiritual spring. It's the act of participating more in the art of life and allowing the elegance of each moment to be brought to the surface. That's a whole different relationship to creativity than what we've been programmed to believe—that we either are somehow allowed to be creative only if we are "good" at whatever the creative act is. That notion is totally constrictive and toxic, and this is why I think it's an important conversation.

Each of us on the planet is part of a movement of energy toward either creativity or destructivity. As humans, we are always doing either one or the other. If we can make our art, our artful life, an addition to the movement of humans waking out of their collective slumber currently on the planet, then there will be more and more of the creative flow toward constructing. This is a major part of this new era—art created out of a generosity toward and for the world.

The creative pulse is very human. In fact, there's an inverted frequency when we're not in an outflow of productivity and creativity. If the natural outflow doesn't happen, the energy that *should* be going out into the world gets inverted into neurosis and tendencies toward lower states of experience like depression and fatigue. So your creativity is a constant that's important to your actual *health*—mentally, physically, and emotionally.

But the creation of dharma art must be harmonic and an outpouring of the meditative mind. Human beauty is found not only in harmony; it is also found in the *creation* of harmony. Creating harmony in everything one sees, feels, touches, or understands is a highly disciplined creative and spiritual act. If you can create only when you feel inspired or you can create only when there is some sort of friction or suffering, then the creative act becomes one of depletion and reinvigoration of suffering, both yours individually and collectively.

The creative act, the act of creation, is happening *constantly* and *consistently* throughout *every single day*, which means that you, as the artist/businessperson/parent/scientist you are, can consistently and constantly tap into it and use it for something fresh. Fresh thought, fresh energy, fresh action. Something truly new and opulent that creates all kinds of moments of kindness and inspiration and deeper humanity on the planet, which makes your art and your life a *different quality of an offering*. It makes your business different. And your parenting different.

DHARMA ART IN ACTION

I really encourage you to take your Invincible Living practices and apply them to your work and life in your own unique and personal way. A transmission happens through this kind of creativity. For truly applied creativity, I believe in getting the body energy moving.

We all have reasons for moving.
I move to keep things whole.

—MARK STRAND

When you move the body, your personal river of energy starts flowing. Then, clarity and inspiration are the orders of the day. This is why I believe that physical yogic practice is inseparable from the true creative pulse.

When it comes down to it, however, you don't have to be a "spiritual artist." As I've said, *all* art done well is deep spiritual practice. There are actually a lot of examples of what I would call dharma art in the contemporary art world right now. It's a growing intersection.

A great example of this is the performance artist Marina Abramović. She's a profound creator who, through the intelligence of her artistry, has accessed spiritual technology. Her piece *The Artist Is Present,* one of her most famous performances, is a completely yogic act, both in intention and in technique. This amazing woman sat for eight hours at a table in the atrium at the Museum of Modern Art in New York City. Visitors were encouraged to sit across from her and look into her eyes. There was no talking, no form of overt communication. Just gazing. This performance continued day after day for three months. There's actually a film about this performance, and it's really quite moving. The amazing part about this piece is that, whether or not Marina Abramović is well versed in ancient yogic techniques, she replicated a very powerful practice and *applied* it. This kind of long-term gazing is called *tratak,* and it's one of the oldest and most potent forms of yogic activation. In the lineage from which I teach, we utilize the tratak in all-day meditation sessions called White Tantric Yoga. And this stuff is *powerful.* One day of White Tantric Yoga is said to equal ten years of daily meditation.

I went to see Marina in a separate piece in 2014, which was also really incredible. There were lines and lines of young people there to see her. So many. And all of these very hip, young, artistic New Yorkers were gathered there to have an art experience, but the art that she does is really a spiritual experience. So everyone there was gathering essentially for a meditative, artistically creative, spiritual experience. And I think this is really profound and *important* because there's a convergence on the planet now. It really doesn't matter if Marina Abramović knows she uses yogic techniques or not. And it doesn't matter what came first. What's significant is that spirituality isn't being relegated to the church or the temple or the mosque or the yoga studio—it's an integrated way of being, thinking, and behaving into all creative acts. And the art world is, organically, turning into a place for human spiritual consciousness to come online. Because being alive in a truly meaningful way is not an "art" technique or "spiritual" technique—it's about *being* human in the most profound and creative of ways.

These practices of art, life, and spirituality are not separate. It is possible to use our meditative practice to enhance sensitivity, to amplify intelligence and originality, and to make something really unique, profound, and activating for people to come into contact with.

You then become an agent for inspiration and your life a spark of fire to light others up with. This is what Yogi Bhajan was describing when he said that the leaders of this new time on the planet would be lighthouses for humanity.

CREATIVE GENIUS

You have the desire to activate and experience your potential for genius, as we all do. That's basic human nature. There is a seed of genius in you. There is a deep desire to tap it and, truly, you *are* meant to awaken it so that you can deliver to the world your very important gifts.

The human system has access to 30 trillion watts of energy, but most of us are running 120. I mean, we're talking major nuclear creative potential here! And this is really one of the simplest antidotes to getting out of habitual human suffering.

An activation of kundalini energy is the source of all real creative genius. That's not to say that Picasso and the Dadaists and everyone weren't deeply entrenched in their suffering. They were. But their *actual* creativity, what made them *truly* great, had nothing to do with their angst. It was the massive kundalini running through them—their connectivity to life and that force of nature moving them to create.

You can see this really well in the artists in history who were considered a little "off." Think of van Gogh, for example. There is so much talk of van Gogh and his mental illness. Really what I believe was going on was that he had a spontaneous kundalini awakening of one sort or another and his nervous system wasn't primed for it. Genius—like love, prosperity, success, and joy—is a high-voltage wave. Suddenly van Gogh was seeing anew and experiencing in full the creative pulse, and he massively, massively tapped into something great and infinite. But his physical system was not able to hold the wattage. And this is something that we see a lot in creatives throughout history.

These techniques to activate the deep ocean of energy and inspiration are also expertly designed to strengthen you to handle these new energies. The kundalini is a door, an access to create out of inspiration and purity. And it's the waking up and amping up of these energies that will take you from commonplace, status quo life to something more extraordinary. Cliché consciousness and the hypnosis of a sleepy life are so seductive. Most of the time, we don't even know that we are doing it until it is too late. Try this simple and profound practice below to begin to wake up and balance your system to receive greater revelation and the energy to do something with it in your day-to-day life.

KIRTAN KRIYA FOR CREATIVE UPLINK

Kirtan Kriya is one of the more famous of the Kundalini Yoga meditations. It uses the mantra *Sa-Ta-Na-Ma*. The sound *Sa* is a sound expression of the Universe. It's like onomatopoeia—only it's quite literal. If you listen to the sound of the Universe, you will hear *Saaaa*. *Ta* is the sound of life. *Na* is the sound of death. *Ma* is the sound of rebirth.

Chanting *Sa-Ta-Na-Ma* is the nuclear form of *Sat Nam* that you were introduced to earlier. Because it is a split of that mantra *Sat Nam*, the *Sa-Ta-Na-Ma* literally has the energy of the atom in it. It's like a mantric atomic bomb. That's why it can do major, major creatively transformative things. Chanting *Sa-Ta-Na-Ma* totally reorganizes your whole thought matrix.

REVELATION AND THE MEDITATIVE SPACE

One of the marks of great creativity is that it offers a revelation to the world in some way. Steve Jobs's great creative act was that he offered the world a system that kept up with the speed of our need to be connected to ourselves and others in a simple and interactive way. Donatella Versace's creative act reveals the beauty of the physical form. Leonardo da Vinci's creative acts reveal the interconnectedness of things.

As humans, we want to grasp a bigger picture of infinity—if not the whole picture. Great artists and yogis get moments of seeing the big picture

CLASSICAL KIRTAN KRIYA

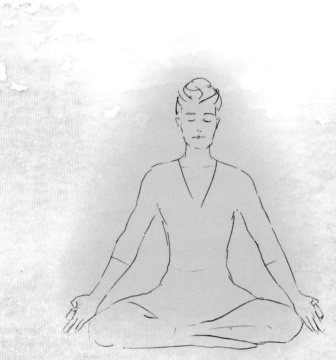

POSTURE: Sit in easy pose.

EYES: Keep your eyes closed, gently focusing up and in at the brow point.

BREATH AND MANTRA: Breathe naturally. Out loud, say each syllable of the mantra *Sa-Ta-Na-Ma* as you alternate touching each finger to the thumb. So on *Sa*, you touch the tip of your index finger to your thumb. On *Ta* you touch your middle finger with your thumb. On *Na* you touch your ring finger. On *Ma*, the pinky finger.

TIME: 3 to 11 minutes

TO END: Inhale, exhale, and relax.

MUDRAS

Mudra means "metaphor." It's a powerful way to adjust the brain. Whenever I'm feeling foggy, I put my hands in a new mudra to restructure the energy and shift my mind.

through either their meditation or their creation. They are trying to show us in the language they know best. The exquisite blend of the finite and infinite *is* art. It also just happens to be the whole reason you're in the human form to begin with.

The fixation on the finite often limits us from accessing infinity in a revelatory way. We get so caught up on the day-to-day and the materiality of life. Because we believe that we are finite beings without the capacity for infinity, we either can't or don't want or are too afraid to look deeper into the infinite.

In reality, our capacity for the infinite is *infinite*. All of the ways that we try to avoid or shirk this experience are just neurotic habits and tendencies that block our creativity. When you use the finite parts of you to relate to the infinite, the creative act becomes more revelatory—in fact, it becomes ecstatic.

The meditative mind is effective for this. There's a way, through our meditative practice, to clean out the subconscious and the finite spaces in us so that the revelation can come through in a powerful way. When we clean the subconscious mind, we create the space for the universal mind, the collective mind, the collective inspiration, or the collective creativity to come through. That establishes a kind of masterful artistry in any area of living—whether you're gardening or loving or parenting or making art.

Many of the revelations of great artists were exactly like this. One of the poet T. S. Eliot's most famous works is *The Waste Land*. But it's a later piece of his art, the *Four Quartets*, that exhibits the revelation of spiritual infinity through the finite forms. He eloquently explores time and space and what is real and what is not. The poems were inspired literally by a spiritual awakening of sorts and compared to *The Waste Land*—where T. S. Eliot was cleaning out his subconscious mind almost literally—his spiritual connectivity is tangible in the *Four Quartets*. Infinity is coming through the structures of the words, sounds, images, and journey. We really get to experience inspiration from the eternal spring rather than from Eliot's finite suffering.

This makes a lot of sense because T. S. Eliot wrote *Four Quartets* toward the end of his life. A lot of times it takes getting toward the end of life, or some finite experience, to be able to have more expansiveness. This is why when people get a medical death sentence of a couple of weeks or months due to illness, they oftentimes feel more alive than ever. All of a sudden, they allow themselves to access their infinite capacity of reality. They finally give themselves permission. What if we had the energy and clarity to access that experience all the time? What kind of experience would be possible for us in the constant unfolding of the miraculous and creative in our lives?

What if instead of waiting for death to come knocking, we accepted and merged with infinity in every moment we could muster of our conscious lives? What if instead of insisting on a fixed, limited, restricted, bounded existence, we could recognize all of reality as part of the perpetual flow? What if? What could happen to our creativity and to the vibrancy of the planet and to the quality and caliber of that vibrancy if we could just stay connected to infinity even a couple of minutes a day?

From the meditative space, the creative pulse begins to become an effective and solid force. Part of the power of this new era is that we have more of the tools and support necessary to create from a space of peaceful, productive beingness. From the vastness: into reality.

"Time present and time past
Are both perhaps present in time future
And time future contained in time past.
If all time is eternally present"

—T. S. ELIOT, *FOUR QUARTETS*

HEARTBEAT MEDITATION FOR EXPANDED VISION

POSTURE: Sit in easy pose. Bring the tips of your index finger and thumb together so that you can feel the pulse of your heartbeat in the tips of your fingers. Lock your front teeth together, tip to tip on top of each other. Press your tongue against your palate.

EYES: Keep your eyes closed, gently focusing up and in at the brow point.

BREATH: Breath is steady, with the focus on the beat of the heart.

TIME: 3 to 11 minutes

TO END: Inhale, exhale, and relax.

CREATIVE ACCOMPLISHMENT

You have the meditative inspiration and the revelation. The ideas are flowing, constant, and consistent, as the creative inspiration is in each moment of living. Now you have to *do it*.

I believe that creative productivity might be the hardest thing for people interested in art and invention. Because it's very easy to have ideas. And it's very fun! You can have an idea and build on that idea and keep building. You can construct a whole realm just within the scope of ideas and thoughts and inspiration. And it can feel like you are really *doing* a lot, because you are *thinking* so much. But we don't want the dreams just to *abound*; we want the dreams to *a-ground*. To take those inspirations out of the ether and into the material realm!

If all of our creativity were just up in the airy-fairy land, nothing would ever change here on earth. In order to make our dreams real in the 3-D, we must break out of the neurotic obsession with the finite and propel into the land of infinite inspiration. Then, you have to be able to come back from the etheric realms and put yourself and your creation into the tangible world. This is slightly more challenging because it requires the bicameral brain. *Bicameral* is a term that refers to the dexterity and ability to use both hemispheres of the brain in harmonic sophistication. We're in a time when we need to have both capacities available to us and we actually *need* to more than ever utilize both hemispheres of our brains.

You can't just be an artist with no business acumen nor can you be a businessperson with no creative pulse. All of these technologies throughout the book are ultimately to make you fully embodied, fully activated, and fully employing your capacities to the best of your ability. And there is not better work in the world than to create models in which others can see their own potential and be inspirited by the possibility of infinity.

Many of these practices I've given develop your capacity to use both sides of the brain. It's very useful to have both logic and intuition, order and randomness, strategy and creative liberation, a dexterous employment of each side of our brain capacity as the moment calls for it.

Let's ground our inspirations in a very real, coherent way that, actually, is very satisfying because it's gratifying to produce. There's a fulfillment when something gets done. And it's important to honor our human need for accomplishment. Accomplishment takes grit, fortitude, and consistency. It took Steve Jobs twelve years between when he was fired—*fired*—from his own company to the time he was brought back on and he revolutionized the world with the iMac. And these were his prime years between the ages of thirty and forty-two. But he didn't give up or stop inventing and being creative.

In the instant-gratification world, it's common that everyone wants to "bitch out" if his or her thing doesn't happen in, like, five seconds. And honestly it is very possible to manifest things very quickly; however, sometimes you don't so the practice of fortitude and patience are deeply powerful. I mean, it took Steve Jobs, a *god* of the technology age, twelve years before his creative genius had matured enough that it was finally ready for fruition. He just stuck

SHORT SET FOR THE BICAMERAL MIND

1. EGO ERADICATOR

NOTES: This short breath exercise balances both hemispheres of the brain, charges the aura, cleanses the blood and lungs, and creates an arc of energy over the head to which the neurology has to respond.

POSTURE: Sit in easy pose. With both hands, curl your fingers so the fingertips are resting on the pads at the base of each finger. Leave your thumbs extended. Stretch your arms up to 60 degrees.

EYES: Keep your eyes closed, gently focusing up and in at the brow point.

BREATH: Do an even and steady Breath of Fire through the nose. Even inhale, even exhale.

TIME: 1 to 3 minutes

TO END: Inhale, hold the breath, stretch your arms up until the thumb tips touch, and stretch the fingers out. Exhale and sweep the arms through the auric field.

2. BRAIN MASSAGE

POSTURE: Continue sitting in easy pose. Gently press the fingertips of both hands together, thumb to thumb, index finger to index finger, and so on.

EYES: Keep your eyes closed, gently focusing up and in at the brow point.

BREATH: Breathe normally. Roll your fingertips around, in and out, as though you are massaging your brain. The fingers correspond to five locations on each side of the brain, so this is very literally what you are doing.

TIME: 1 to 3 minutes

TO END: Inhale, exhale, and relax.

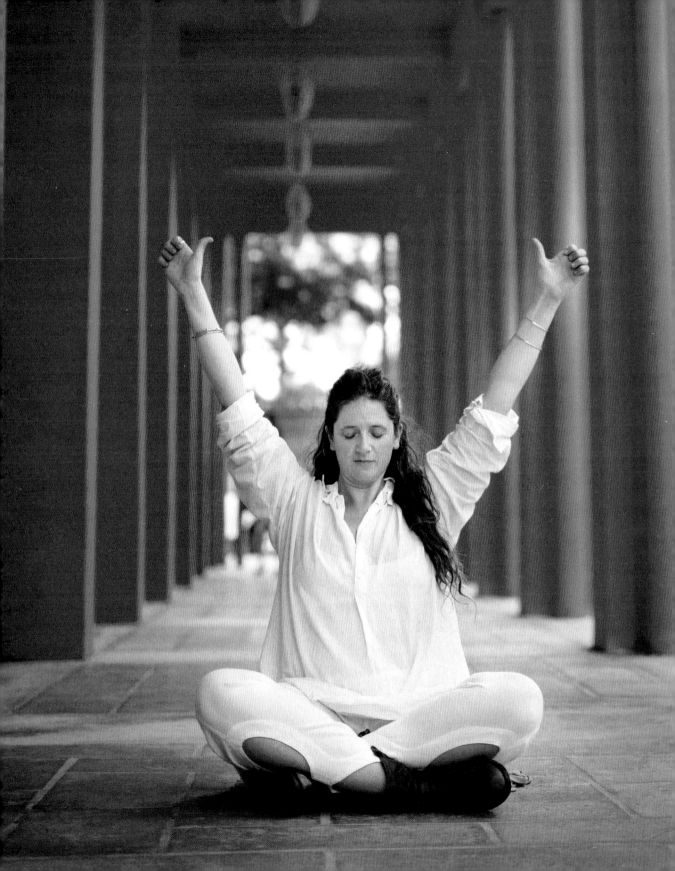

to the infinite revelation that people wanted technology that was *elegant,* that was art. He kept his eye on the ball.

True art calls for fortitude—fortitude and focus. Now, that doesn't have to be scary. We don't have to go from the beautiful land of infinite inspiration and then slave drive ourselves into productivity. That kills the inspiration. We just need focus. We need to get up every day, grab the inspiration, and then, step by step, do the work.

One of my favorite techniques for focus is the rishi knot because it's very sensory and simple, not to mention ever so hip right now.

RISHI KNOT TECH

If you need a certain amount of consolidation—if you need to do something that requires a certain amount of brain concentration—wrap your hair into a bun right on top of your crown, also called the anterior fontanel. This is the bonus for both men and women growing their hair out. Hair conducts solar energy, and the anterior fontanel, this part of the skull that used to be soft when we were babies, is a place of great cosmic and solar transmission. When you wrap your hair there and tie it in a rishi knot, you focus and consolidate more solar energy into this center. This makes you very aware, attentive, and skillful in your decisions and actions throughout the day.

The rishi knot stimulates the fontanel and activates the two solar centers on either side of the fontanel, creating a three-pronged crown of electricity. So this is very good technology for creativity and productivity.

Creativity is the cure. It's medicine and it will heal and reveal you to you in ways that nothing else will. May you become a genius of your own life and may each day be the most ultimate creative act of living, being, and loving.

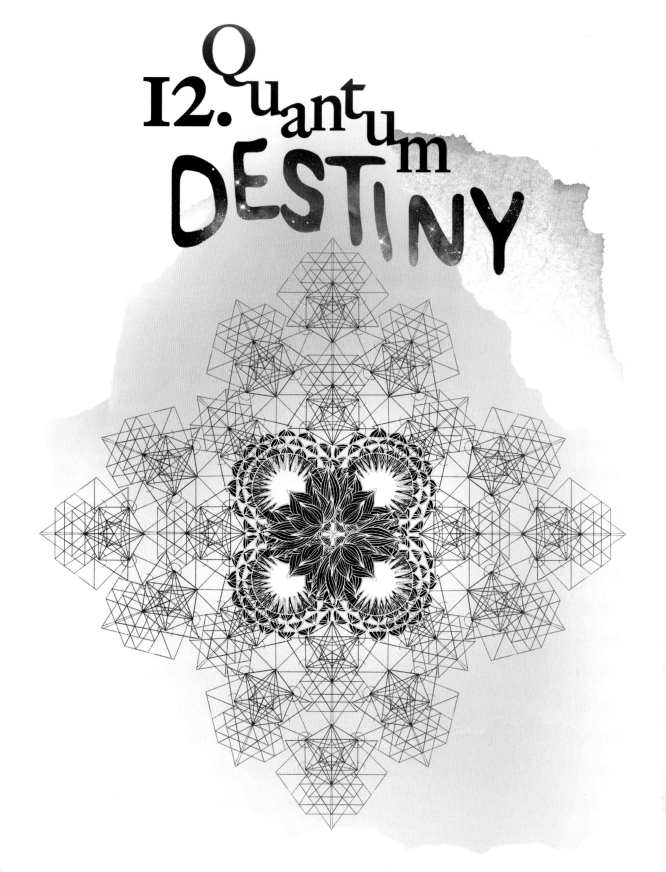

12. Quantum DESTINY

There is a destiny for you. A fulfillment of your purpose. A high frequency for your total life experience.

Kundalini Yoga puts—and keeps—you in charge of your own destiny. In the past, your destiny patterns, your karma, were considered set and a place of disempowerment.

This is one of the major advances of Kundalini Yoga and Meditation. The yogic, bioenergetic technology of Kundalini Yoga is so precise, so cultivated in its accuracy, that just a simple eleven-minute meditation can shift lifetimes of patterning. In the past, when maybe you'd have had to spend your whole existence working off a bad karma, you now have the power to reorganize your thoughts and therefore your experience of reality. Through Kundalini Yoga, you can activate *destiny* for greater fulfillment in this lifetime, and learn to hack the mainframe to reprogram any thought or behavior that is keeping you from this.

You no longer have to take the long way around. You don't have to suffer for centuries upon centuries—

or even years upon years or months upon months. You can change your experience right now, in a matter of minutes.

CLEARING THE CONFUSION

While we have an intuitive sense about our destinies, there's also a lot of confusion around what destiny means and how to live it. Many people, once they find some spiritual path, get this idea that they're not supposed to do the job that they currently do. Their work is beneath them in some way. They just can't handle the water-cooler chat. It's not their "destiny." This is a real misconception. Yogic practice says very strongly that if you want anything to change in your life, you have to have enough energy to find beauty and elegance in the most mundane of tasks and bring that up to the surface of your experience. It's a highly meditative and spiritually disciplined task to do that, especially if you don't like what you do for work or who you have to do it with.

Whatever is already here, whatever job you have, whatever relationship you have, whatever chore you have to do, do it with openness and with the inherent beauty of the moment and the people—then you will open up almost instantaneously. In the West, everything always looks much greener on the other side. We don't want to engage with what's in front of us. We've been programmed to consume, always looking for the next better thing. But if we train ourselves to serve and engage in each moment, literally we become evolution in action.

Your job is not a block to your destiny. Waking up in some way in your ordinary life is actually such a wonderful opportunity to engage in a bigger way with everything through a more actualized version of yourself. This means that you don't get on a high horse or embody the classic spiritual self-righteousness. You may leave your job eventually, but you're definitely not too spiritual for it. The true concept of destiny is ultimately vibrating and broadcasting the biggest, most compassionate version of yourself. You can do that anywhere—in line at the grocery, dealing with the public, writing an email, or cooking dinner.

Many things are currently changing in our society and consciousness, and therefore there is a breaking out of some of the programming of what success used to look like. Some are still locked into the model of existence to go to college, get the thing, then do the thing, and then do that thing for the rest of your life and then retire. Or the model to elevate money, money, money at the expense of living. That's not truly a fulfillment of destiny and will always leave you empty-handed no matter how shiny and seductive it was. And no matter how ordinary the task is, if our intention is to become more alive in each moment and each day, then whatever it is will become deeply satisfying.

Destiny gives you the heights of living.

The ways that we give our gifts are changing. Every five years, even every two years, people are redefining themselves. This is good news. There's an alignment with bigger truths of ourselves. That doesn't mean you should drop your 3-D world the moment you have some wink of spiritual energy or experience. But it also doesn't mean staying put in a place that doesn't allow you to expand into the fullest experience of your incarnation. As you engage more deeply with what's in front of you, you will graduate in some sense, and new opportunities and calibers of experience will be available to you.

You may not know what your destiny is exactly. That's okay. First we want to lock in a deeper resonance of fulfillment and happiness, because once we have that experience in our beingness, then it starts to illuminate right action more and more clearly. Clarity and joy have momentum.

DESTINY DISCOVERY

We know two things: if you engage deeper in *love* with what is in front of you, *something* will be revealed. That's number one. Number two is that if you *serve* more than just your own personal preferences in this era, then something's going to open up that's a higher frequency of the destiny.

When you don't know why you're here, you just have one mandate and it's actually quite simple! In every moment of every day, you create more prayer, more *love,* and more genuine interaction between human beings, and you see where that takes you. This energy will open up the chambers of your destiny and, ultimately, the powerfully magnetic energy of your heart. Bringing more love into every interaction on the planet—and treating every moment as a prayer in action, a self-blessing—will automatically start to give you more direction into destiny, purpose, and mission.

TIME STREAMS

There are literally boundless destiny streams available to you. If there are a thousand thoughts in the blink of an eye and two ionic poles to each thought, and each thought is a choice that takes on a new destiny stream, there are literally exponentially more options with each decision you make. And the choices you don't make keep streaming, whether you are aware of them or not, whether you're on their wave of reality or not.

Yogi Bhajan had some beautiful and powerful teachings around the time streams of destiny and the time streams of fate. There are multiple levels, multiple realities simultaneously happening. As I explained earlier, it truly is like a Choose Your Own Adventure book. You read up to a certain point in the book, and if you want to go down the forest path, flip to page sixty-three, and if you want to continue on the paved road, keep reading.

These options of fate and destiny are not subtle. They're actually quite concrete. Even though we're not attuned to them, even though we're not taught about them, you can always actually feel different timelines of possibility.

Such timelines are very tangible and navigable. We all have dreams, visions, and missions. Part of the challenge and the *joy* of living is figuring out how you are going to pursue and accomplish your dreams, visions, and missions—how you're going to get through obstacles. And how you're going to make this journey with the fewest stubbed toes and scraped knees as possible. Also the fewest casualties in your wake. When you want to navigate this life with success, and I mean really navigate, not just numb out and follow the hypnotic cookie-cutter unfulfilled protocol, then you have to learn to be sensitive. You become aware of the variables and then sophisticated enough to move with them.

It takes energy to maneuver through all of the possibilities and to not mis-take. Energy and *command*.

COMMANDING TIME STREAMS

We live on a polarity planet. Everything has a double termination, an electromagnetic duality inherent in our human experience. And *fate* is an uncontrolled relationship with that duality. Fate is our lack of command, our lack of mastery of this elemental duality.

When you are not in command, it means the wave hits you and takes you. Sometimes you're happy; sometimes you're sad. Sometimes you're in the mix and everything is going well. In the next moment, nothing is going right and you can't figure out how things fell apart or what to do next. You're at the whim of time. And that is commonly just called a life.

Destiny is a mastered relationship with this duality. You command the charge of time and space. The polarity is a given, but *you* direct the sequence of the polarities. So instead of being at a disastrous work party till 3:00 A.M. and then not being able to find a cab home and waking up on the wrong side of the bed the next day, you direct a different experience. One that is more to your liking. Or even better, one that is more to your satisfaction and fulfillment. When you have that command and that dexterity, you are beginning to live destiny.

One of my favorite applications of this command is called Making a Mold of the Day. Here's how it works.

MAKING A MOLD OF THE DAY

DIRECTIONS: In the morning, take a survey of the tasks you have to do that day: what you have to engage in, what you have to be accountable for—everything. Then make some determinations about how you're going to spend the energy of your day. You create a *mold* of how you want your day to be. Then you put your day into the mold.

This is *not* what we normally do. Normally we wake up on the wrong side of the bed, we're trying to catch up, and we let the day run us. This is different.

You create a *directional* mold of the day and then put your day into that mold. This will give you power as well as security and steadiness to make decisions and be clear minded and focused.

RADIANT BODY

The time of the hustle and the hassle is over. We have been highly conditioned to believe that the hustle is the only way to make it. The hustle and all of the energy thereof actually gets in the *way* of your destiny.

There is an opportunity now to activate your radiant and magnetic consciousness. When you do this, you activate what we yogically call the radiant body. All who are supposed to meet you, all opportunities meant to be yours, all situations that you want to experience, will come to you. It is a part of the magnetic law of the Universe.

Now, you do have to *work and show up*. And I mean that in all senses of the word *work*. You have to be willing and attentive. You have to practice—hence all the little treasures of practices I've given you in this book that have been gifted to me by my teachers. But the time of the hustle mentality is over.

Deactivating the hustle instinct can take a little bit of work. We're getting more and more sensitive as humans, so any way you are wired toward the hustle—and these wirings can be very subtle—you can train yourself to start noticing. Just get intuitive about how you hustle and how you compromise or prostitute yourself for something externally driven.

I know this is very foreign to our programming, but if you want to have a greater flow of energy exchange, such as more cash in exchange for products, you don't have to "advertise." You don't need to convince or persuade or trick anybody into buying. You don't have to hustle by fixating on your social media likes. What will make you attract the most incredible experiences of your destiny is completely and committedly having a practice of clearing yourself to be a living example of what it means to be *comfortable* being yourself. Look around—all the most successful people in history had some sort of radiant power through their own comfort of being themselves one way or another. When you have this, it makes you someone who people *want* to be around or listen to or buy services from and so on. This is a very tangible result of your yogic and radiant body practice.

People want energy, because at a basic level, it takes energy to live some version of your destiny. So the more you can practice and generate energy, the easier it is to navigate the time and space of your most elevated life.

Now, we do live in a time when people are still under the influence of major hypnotic advertising, social media loops, and other collective distraction propaganda. But that time is fading. People are by the moment getting more sensitive. So don't get caught in that loop. It will soon be outdated, and you will wonder why things aren't working out for you.

The impression you make and the impression you leave are the projective essence of your radiant body and aura. When you use your radiant body to achieve and energetically leap into higher vibrations of your destiny, things can happen really fast. And I mean *really* fast! And if it doesn't happen really fast for you, don't lose hope and retreat back into the hustle, defeated. Sometimes it takes a little time to establish the auric and radiant body architecture. So just stand up, command again. It's there, and it's yours to claim. You wouldn't have dreamed it or imagined it if it somehow wasn't a possibility of your destiny. Again, patience pays. Alertness pays. Practice reveals your perfection and the perfection of the moment.

ENERGY

So to develop radiance and to command the mold of your day, you need *energy*. And another way of saying that is, you need conviction, assurance, and commitment.

When you have self-doubt or a lack of energy, that survives on one type of thought form: *There is something inherently wrong with me.* Unfortunately, this root insecurity is still weighing on the human mind today, maybe heavier than ever. The base of it is lodged into our psyches through the religious teachings on original sin. The capitalist agenda based on our own insecurity makes a lot of money off of us thinking there is something wrong with us.

There's a major investment in having people believe that *there is not enough* and *you are not enough*. When you doubt yourself, you are low energy, and when you are low energy, you are more controllable, and when you are more controllable, you are more exploitable for money and all other kinds of things. This is really noxious because just one thought form of self-doubt instantaneously takes 30 percent of your energy for the day. That's a lot: *30 percent*! So self-doubt is a place of massive energy loss. If you want to change your destiny, you have to start to understand that you really can't afford that habitual belief of unworthiness or self-doubt.

It takes some strength and some yogic training to stand up and say, "Okay, not only do I believe that I am enough and that I can handle this and that I'm worthy of it, but I'm also going to step into it . . . even if I don't know what I'm doing." But remember this: not only is there nothing wrong with you, but you are also the most powerful creation that ever was created.

This is why "Fake it till you make it" is actually such a deep spiritual practice. Every time you take that leap of faith, even if you don't know what you are doing, you build an energetic ladder to another level of yourself. When you act with faith in yourself and with conviction, you start to seal up the spots where energy had been leaking away from you. To start to believe in your destiny, or even just to engage with a higher frequency of your life on this planet, these practices help to create a tighter container of energy and seal up and heal the places we have been leaky.

GUILT, COMPLAINT, AND LINEAL HABITS

It's time we really cut the guilt. Guilt is a big waste of energy and is another way we leak a lot of our command of our lives. Spiritual guilt is a whole new renaissance of guilt. I see it a lot because when people find a spiritual practice, they all of a sudden transfer a lot of their religious and societal guilt onto their spiritual practice. They didn't do the meditation, or they did but not for as long as they think they should have. Spiritual practice is a *great* place to put all of your guilt consciousness. And it's very seductive that way, because we have a lot of guilt in our lineages and a lot of guilt that's running through the collective consciousness. It doesn't serve any sort of your progression to lose energy on these different incarnations of guilt.

Another way we quickly lose our intuitive and action power is through complaining. It's a highly effective practice to cut down on the amount of complaining you do. Literally one complaint closes 30 percent of our intuitive faculties like an iron gate. That's 30 percent on top of the 30 percent we've already lost from self-doubt. You can see how this quickly snowballs into fatigue, confusion, and misdirection.

We picked up many of these mental and psychoemotional habits through our lineage and early childhood programming. Kundalini Yoga is a *raj* yoga—a royal path and lineage. The raj of your experience is a self-concept that is based in your own blessing of yourself. This is the teaching of the raj yoga: *There's a throne. It's there for you. The only person who can enthrone you is you. The throne is your destiny. The throne is waiting for you to be brave enough to be you.*

So many habits are deeply ingrained, you might wonder how exactly you are going to put a stop to the ones that have continued the last seven generations of your family to enthrone yourself in your rightful place. Almost any practice I've shared in this book will do it. It doesn't have to be complicated—as mythic and poetic as it sounds, it can literally be just you—through the couple of minutes you've committed a day—paving a path to the experience of your own human excellence and majesty.

SELF-BLESSING

Most of our self-concepts were created in the womb under circumstances beyond our control. These self-concepts were not the highest accord, order, or vibration. Then, throughout our lives, we've engaged in a lot of negative refer-

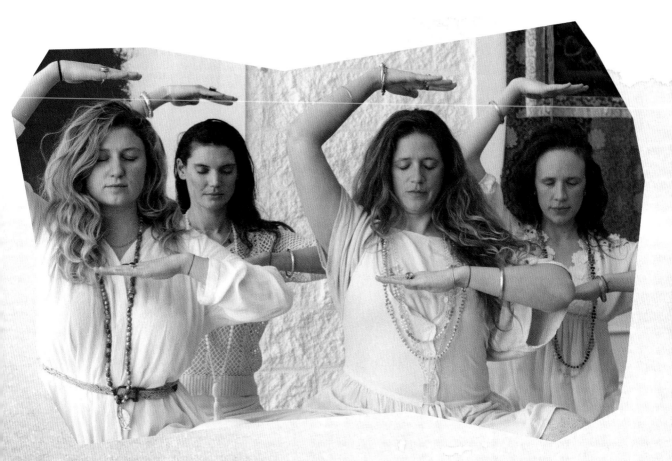

MEDITATION FOR SELF-BLESSING

POSTURE: Sit in easy pose. Place your right hand 6 inches above the crown of your head with the palm facing down. Bend your left elbow parallel to the ground to hold your left hand at the level of your heart, palm down.

EYES: Keep your eyes closed, gently focusing up and in at the brow point.

BREATH AND MANTRA: Breathe naturally and chant in monotone: *I bless myself, I bless myself, I bless myself. I am, I am.*

TIME: 3 minutes

TO END: Inhale, hold the breath, repeat the mantra mentally, and exhale. Repeat twice. Relax.

encing about ourselves—like *What a piece of crap I am*—from every subsequent trauma, embarrassing mishap, or whatever else we might have gone through: social exclusion, critical teachers, or fighting or busy parents. We take on so many negative and destructive self-concepts, it actually takes *a lot* of training and patience to reprogram our concepts of ourselves.

One of the basic parts of that training is blessing yourself. This is a daily process. From the moment you wake up till the moment you go to sleep for the night, you learn to bless yourself. I can tell you now, it's a rigorous spiritual practice—one of the deepest.

I really invite you to practice this: *Bless my body, bless the work I'm doing, bless my partner, bless my family, bless, bless, bless.* This mantra helps you reprogram your self-concept, which gives you the kind of successful feedback loop that will create self-reverence—one that is solid, secure, and ultimately beneficial for all of humanity.

DAILY PRACTICE

It's very easy to get tossed around in and by life. But we are not here to be shaken by time; we are here to shake time. This is the difference. This is Invincible Living.

Human integrity is above time and space. We are not meant to be swallowed by time and space. This is the basic lesson of human life given by Yogi Bhajan, "Humans *make* time and *give* grace to space." But in order to do this, we have to master time and space. The way that we make time is through the relationship with our mind, and the way that we cultivate a relationship with our mind is through our meditation *practice*.

> *Meditation, it is between You and Now,*
> *You and your Destiny.*
>
> —YOGI BHAJAN

I've included dozens of yogic breath practices, meditations, affirmations, diets, and lifestyle practices in this book. If you pick just *one* of them to do on a daily basis, to become a master of, your practice will create a vortex of momentum, or wind horse, as they call it in Tibetan Buddhism, to propel you into higher, more integrated realms of your consciousness and destiny.

You don't have to wait. You don't have to work for decades. You don't have to self-flagellate for success. With enough energy in your system, your ten bodies *know* how to navigate more successfully. Because the ten bodies are naturally attuned to radiance, they will—with the proper energy—instinctively allow your natural skills and intelligence to determine right action and move in it. All of the ten bodies are balanced and activated through the yogic breaths, meditations, affirmations, diets, and lifestyle technology outlined throughout this book.

Daily practice doesn't need to be done like some sort of religious ritual. It can be fresh and alive, an act of self-discipleship and discipline that allows you to trust your commitment to fulfilled living more and more deeply. Daily practice grants you a victory over your tiredness, your sluggishness, your fatigue, your challenges and laziness.

There's actually a physical biochemistry to staying steadfast, secure, contained, conscious, and relaxed. By practicing Kundalini Yoga every day, you create that physiology. You set the biochemical foundation for long-term prosperity, health, and vitality on a daily basis—with just a couple of minutes of practice. So the times when your practice feels tough, when everything wants to magnetically pull you from doing it . . . that's when the

Science of Angles

Kundalini Yoga is a science of angles and triangles. And different body angles have unique physical and energetic effects on the body.

Keeping my arms at 60 degrees increases lung capacity. It also opens up heart meridian and triggers the flow of compassion.

Angles of Legs

0–6 inches—heals ovaries and reproductive organs
6–18 inches—strengthens navel point and kidneys
1–2 feet—cleanses liver, spleen, gallbladder, and pancreas
1.5–2.5 feet—detoxes upper stomach
2–3 feet—develops heart and lungs
Over 4 feet—stimulates thyroid, parathyroid, and pineal glands
90°—feeds pineal and pituitary glands, and memory

I wake up during the ambrosial hours (3:00 A.M. to 6:00 A.M.) to practice two and a half hours of yoga before sunrise. During this time, the angle of the sun to the Earth creates a very sacred space and the efforts of my yoga practice are forty times more powerful.

Balancing my lower triangle (the first three chakras) with upper triangle (the heart, throat, and third eye chakras) gives a complete sense of embodiment.

To Polaris

Equator

work is even more valuable. That's when it's not necessarily blissful or pretty but just real. When you *still* do it, those are the moments of true alchemical transformation in you.

It is nice to get up and do your practice as soon as you wake. This really sets the energetic tone and current for the day. And you can feel the difference throughout the whole day. All of a sudden, your day just starts running smoother. Things become synchronistic, and you have all kinds of successes, big and small, that lead to a satisfying experience of your day.

There are a few of us real fanatics out there who get up at around three or four in the morning and do our yoga practice at that hour. From the 3:00 to 6:00 A.M. window, there is something called the Amrit Vela, or ambrosial hours. And it's a powerful time to practice because any yoga set or meditation you do during this window is amplified fortyfold in your body-mind system. If your daily practice is like depositing a thousand dollars into your energetic bank, practicing it during those hours is like depositing the same amount of money and then the bank multiplies it to forty thousand dollars—so it's a good return on investment.

But whenever or wherever you practice, and for however long—the very act of those couple of minutes may be the greatest gift you've ever given yourself, because in essence, you are giving your self back to your self. It is a great, great treasure that you are uncovering, one that you have not even scratched the surface of, even if you are already a profound yogic and meditative practitioner. It is *infinite*. You are *infinite*.

There's no pressure here and no indoctrination, but the benefits of Kundalini Yoga are cumulative. You can spend your energy money really fast, but if you practice daily, you always have something for that crazy, shit storm of a day. Additionally, a lot of times we're building new habits or breaking old ones that need daily reaffirmation, so it doesn't matter if you get up at the break of dawn or if you do your practice for three minutes or three hours, if you are consistent, you will make great strides! And when you miss, you just keep going. No drama, no guilt. Just a long, wide road of incredible human experience in front of you. Train your mind to always see the big picture and your little burp won't fall into the pattern of what often happens, which is where people get so guilty and heavy-handed with themselves that they never meditate again.

Now, consistency is no easy task. About 80 to 90 percent of the time, you do your practice because you *have* to, not because you want to. Very rarely at first do you ever *want* to do your practice every day.

Kundalini Yoga is a technology that will make you happy, healthy, and holy, but that doesn't mean it will be easy. Even if your daily practice is nothing more than just doing the Breath for Victory I gave in the first chapter of this book, something in you will still resist doing it. That practice is so easy and really enjoyable, but there's going to be that *one* day when your subconscious mind convinces you not to do it or the day when you just "forget." That's natural. But that's the day that, if you can catch it, you do it anyway and create grit and begin to really trust yourself. It's quite beautiful.

There are so many forces reminding you again and again of failure, misfortune, misery, and mistakes. Make it a point every day to saturate yourself in something positive, the higher frequencies, so you create a rhythm where you are moving faster than the hypnosis of negativity, comparison, violence, and gluttonous consumerism.

So when you practice daily, on a consistent basis, it creates an angle to your life that gives you a major amount of energy, which gives you power and choice. This brings your light to the surface. When you win, when you succeed over that insidious self-sabotage riptide, that victory will serve you for the rest of the day and truly for more than you can even know or fathom.

So here's the basic formula for a daily practice. It can get a whole lot fancier than this, and you can also really adjust it to your lifestyle—meaning you just do your practice wherever, whatever way you can. However, this is a pretty basic, doable framework.

VERY BASIC DAILY PRACTICE

1. Wake up. Say something positive to yourself or inhale *Sat,* exhale *Nam.*

2. Go to the bathroom, brush your teeth, and splash some cold water on your face.

3. Find a quiet spot to meditate where you know you will not be disturbed.

4. Tune in. Say the mantra *Ong Namo Guru Dev Namo* three times.

5. Begin your practice. Your practice can be as short as a three-minute meditation to however long you would like it to be. A "full" practice would be:

   A. Pranayam

   B. A yoga set

   C. Meditation

   However, feel free to just do one of these as your personal practice.

6. Relax for a moment before you close out your practice and seal it with a long *Sat Nam.*

Feel free to adjust this formula to your lifestyle. As I wrote in the first chapter, the point of yoga is not to be a "good" yogi or a "bad" yogi. It's to have an *experience.* And my intention for your experience of daily practice is this: bioenergetically, daily practice is a place where you create yourself and your reality for several moments each day—a place where you can tune up, tune in, and get ready to be the most stellar version of yourself possible.

So whether that practice is a cold shower, a strong yoga set, or a meditation that you don't want to do, you're basically making your system get stronger. Daily practice is not comfortable. Nor should it be. But it gives you the conviction to know that you can do anything and face anything—any stress, any strain. *You already woke up and you already won.*

> *If a person in the morning does not move his body in such a way that the capacity of his body developed during his sleeping hours is not activated to take away the stress and strain of the day, then we are getting right straight into a problem for the whole day. We will think that we are awake, that we are perfect ba ba ba, but it doesn't work out that way.*
>
> —YOGI BHAJAN

Basically, a lot of healing happens during sleep. However, if you don't get up and direct the energy in a certain way, then the healing that happened during sleep doesn't know how to be utilized properly. So you can say to yourself, "I am a perfect being, a child of God, an instrument of the Universe . . ." or whatever love and light nonsense you want, but it doesn't work out that way unless you *practice*!

That's why the main mantra for the Aquarian Age, the main wave of the mind, is *Keep up*. Keep up because the world is changing and we have to get stronger as quickly as we can.

The subconscious mind, and all of its quagmires, has a particular pace,

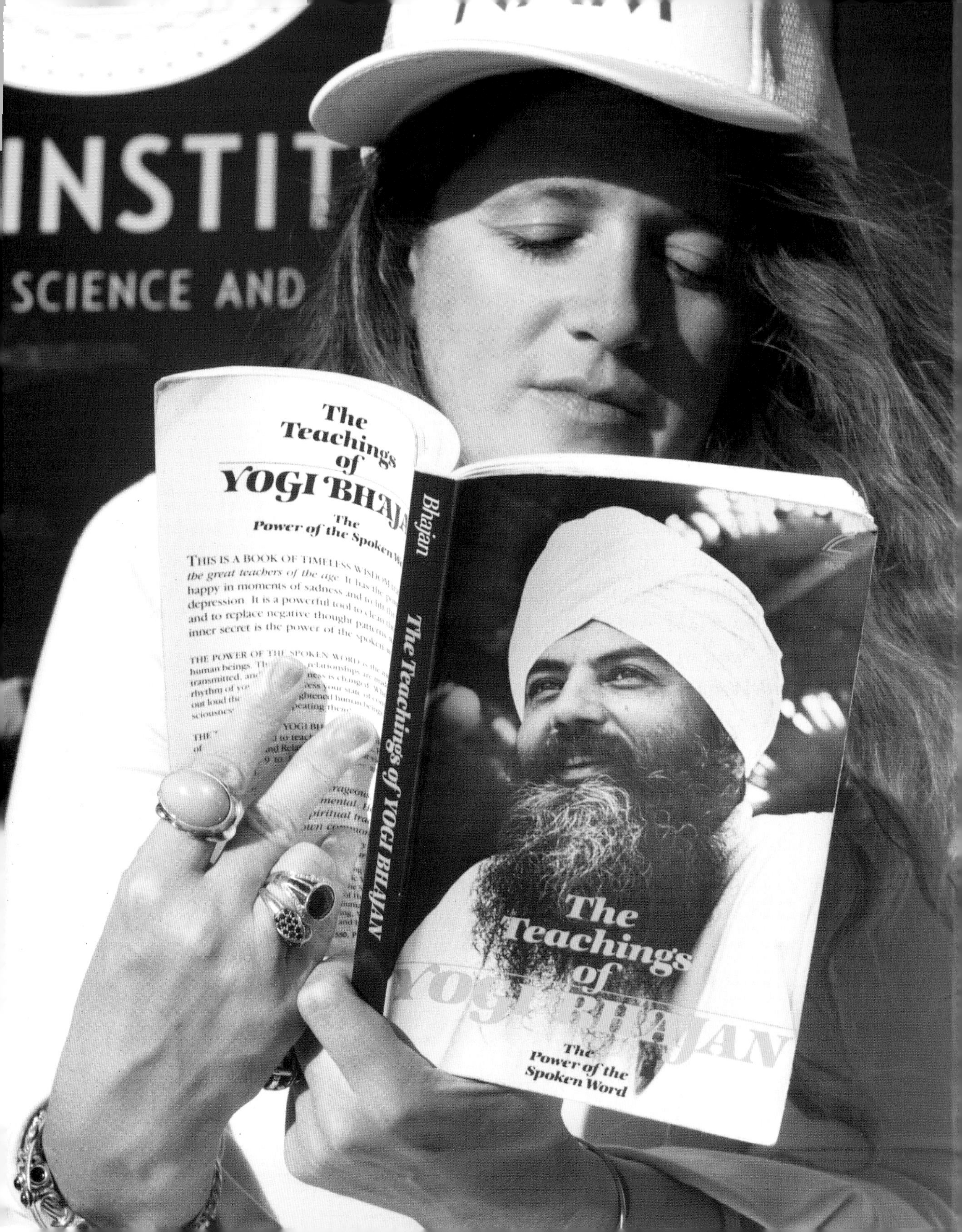

so we use the movement, or kriya, we use the mudra, we use the sound current, we use the mantra to create a velocity in us that is literally faster than the speed of neurosis and unhappiness. And that velocity will catapult you beyond the pace of these subconscious quagmires—the habits of self-hatred and self-loathing. Personal practice gives you a running start—you catch the day before the day catches you.

If you want to know who you are, if you really want to know who you are, if you want to know *where* you are, meaning a kind of litmus test of what's going on with you, if you want to know how you are, where to go, and how to get there, the practice is to keep up. Keep up no matter what's happening in your life. And when you don't want to keep up, use the resistance, in a kind of yogic aikido countermove, to create *more* energy, *higher* velocity, and a *longer* trajectory.

Invincible Living is a daily choice to keep up, to find your basic sanity, to express it through creative and compassionate choices, and to maintain it through consistent, no-nonsense practice. This equation of awakened life will grant you access to a level of human experience that is unfathomably more fulfilling than what we've been told is possible. It will give you strength and courage to find some piece of the mystery of yourself and give it to the world with generosity, energy, and abandon. Truly being invincible is conducting a life whose keystone is clarity of mind, generosity of action and creativity, and not being afraid to actually *live*—with all the pitfalls, failures, successes, expansions, and contractions thereof. There is dignity and divinity in living this way, and may you use these invincible technologies of Kundalini Yoga and Meditation to create the kind of society and world that we know is possible.